102Challenges

Become the Best You

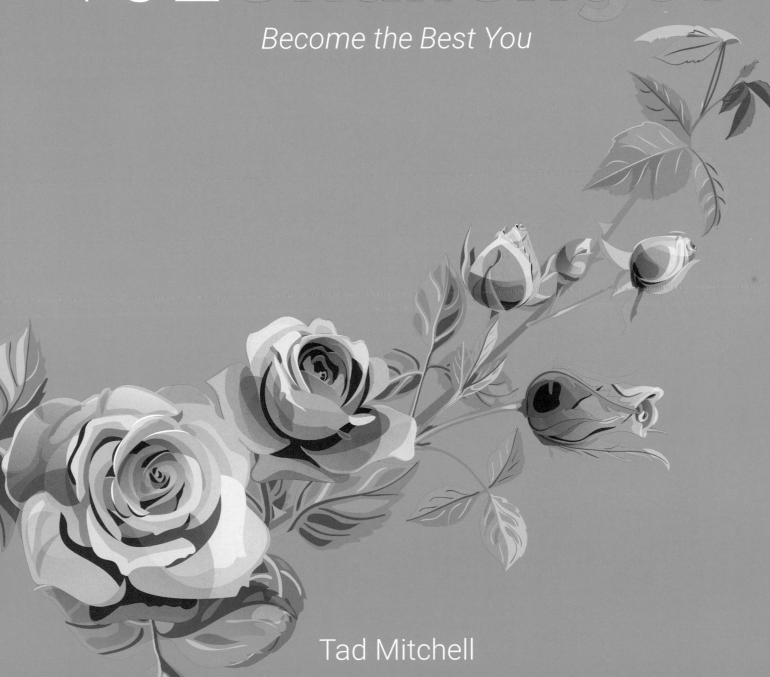

Tad Mitchell

Thank you to the WellRight team who served as guinea pigs testing the challenges. Thank you to Renee and Tricia, our editors. Thank you to our reviewers. Thank you to Tamara who refined the artwork and did the layout. Thank you to all who provided feedback.

Tad

Disclaimer: Information in 102 Challenges is for educational purposes only and is not meant to substitute for the advice of a medical professional. You should consult with a health care professional before starting any diet, exercise, or supplementation program.

First Edition

Printed in U.S.A.

ISBN 978-0-9964417-5-9

More information about the book can be found at www.102Challenges.com.

Reviewers

Medical

David Mitchell, MD, PhD

Nutrition

Kristen Balchan, RD, LDN

Exercise

Michael Grimsley, MPH, CHES, CSCS

Psychology

Christian Laplante, PhD, R PSYCH, MFT

Financial

Cherrish Holland, Certified Credit Counselor
Brian Ramaker, Certified Financial Advisor, AAMS®

Foreword

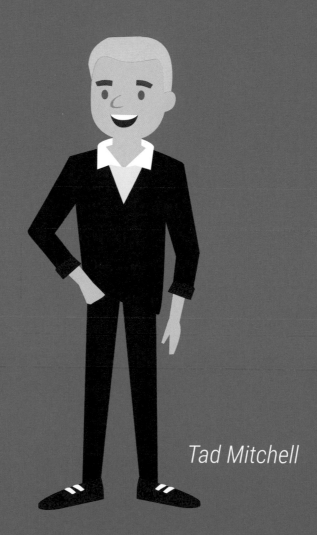

Tad Mitchell

I'm delighted to be writing another challenge book. With the help of everyone at WellRight, we were able to come up with another 102 challenges. In this second book, we pushed beyond the traditional dimensions of wellness (physical, emotional, social, and financial) into other realms to include occupational wellness and purpose.

I say "we" because everyone at WellRight (including our customers and partners) has helped come up with these ideas. Each month, we pilot four or more challenges to see how they work. Some don't work well and we remove them from the list; we adjust others so they work better. The experimentation always leads to new ideas.

In challenging ourselves to become better, a warm vibe permeated throughout our organization. Sure, we've had bumps in the road and every day isn't perfect, but the general trend has been moving us in a very positive direction. Our employees enjoy working together, productivity is increasing, and everyone is generally happy. Former employees return occasionally because they miss the close-knit family feeling in our office.

Historically, corporate wellness has focused on health care cost savings—an important and achievable goal. However, wellness within a company can be so much more than that. It's the perfect platform to help employees become better people. In turn, better people make better organizations—generating returns that are far greater than those of a traditional wellness program.

If an organization tried to educate its employees on how to be happier or how to treat co-workers better, it wouldn't work. Rather, companies can have a wellness program that awards points for activities like listing things you are grateful for or complimenting your co-workers. Such activities accomplish the same goal but do so in a self-driven, gamified format. Imagine how successful and enjoyable your organization could be with happier and kinder employees. Challenge them to become better and see where your company can go!

Introduction

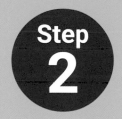
Step 1
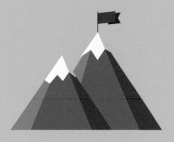
Ask yourself what you should work on

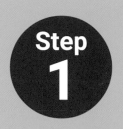
Step 2

Challenge yourself to try it for 30 days

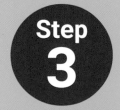
Step 3
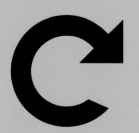
Repeat for the rest of your life

We are all born with an innate desire to become better. Then life happens. The list of things we'd like to do better is very long, and we have so much going on that we settle for merely good enough. As we struggle to keep up with life, we tell ourselves that we are doing the best we can. In reality, we become stagnant, always striving for more but progressing toward "better" at a very slow rate—mildly disappointed that we are not fulfilling our inner desire to progress.

It doesn't have to be that way. You can become better at a quicker pace and keep up with life at the same time. In fact, you actually need the rigors of life to make this pursuit possible. The solution lies in listening to your thoughts and impressions and then submitting to what your heart tells you. However, this is much easier said than done.

Ask yourself what is one thing you need to work on to become a better person. Sometimes meditation can help to clear your mind so you can see more clearly. Other times you may get the answer to this question when you are going full speed in life. The trick is discerning between the right answer and random thoughts. If you find yourself forcing an idea or thinking it through logically repeatedly, you may be on the wrong track. Conversely, if you feel at peace with the idea, like it just fits, then you're probably on the right track.

Next, turn that improvement idea into a challenge. It can be a challenge from this book, a slight variation, or something entirely new. Always listen to your heart. It will let you know where to start. When you craft your challenge, it should have some key elements. It should be simple, achievable, clearly defined, encourage daily activity, allow for exceptions, have a set duration, and be trackable. (See *101 Challenges: Become the Best You* for more details on designing challenges.)

Complete your challenge and then repeat the process. Your heart may tell you to keep working on the same thing or to move on to something else. Over time you will find yourself progressing at lightning speed. Initially the things your heart tells you to work on may not make sense, but eventually they will weave together to make you a new, happier person—and a much more powerful force for good in the world.

Purpose

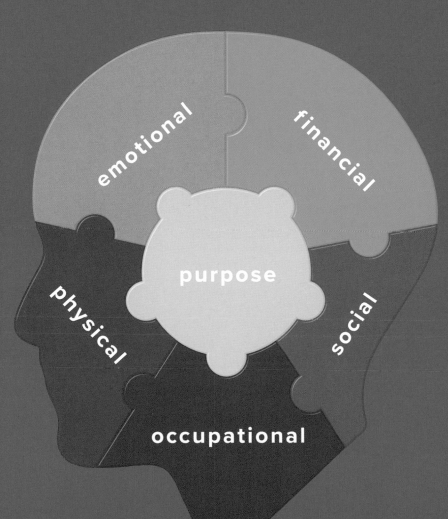

emotional

financial

physical

purpose

social

occupational

Purpose is what holds all the dimensions of wellness together. If you don't have a purpose, why would you do anything?

I have a friend who tried to quit smoking. I was concerned and asked her some questions to try to help: "How many cigarettes do you smoke now? How many did you used to smoke? Where do you get your cigarettes?" Then I had the thought to ask her why she wanted to quit. Without hesitation she replied that she wanted to quit so she could be there for her teenage son (both her parents had died at her age, one from smoking-related problems). That's the power of purpose!

If you don't have a personal mission statement, take the Mission Possible Challenge and create one. If you need inspiration to come up with one, take the Gift List Challenge and ask 10 people what your gifts are. Once you have created your personal mission statement, take the True North Challenge and ponder your personal mission statement each day. Finding your purpose and trying to live in accordance with it will change how you approach life—and leave you more satisfied with your life than you've ever been before.

With neither purpose nor direction, we are like a boat that's tossed about by the waves, with no course nor aim. With purpose and direction, we still experience waves in our lives, but we know our destination and will progress on our journey.

It is my sincere hope the concepts presented in this book will help you better enjoy your journey through life, and that having your purpose in hand may help you become the person you want to be faster than ever before. Are you up for a challenge?

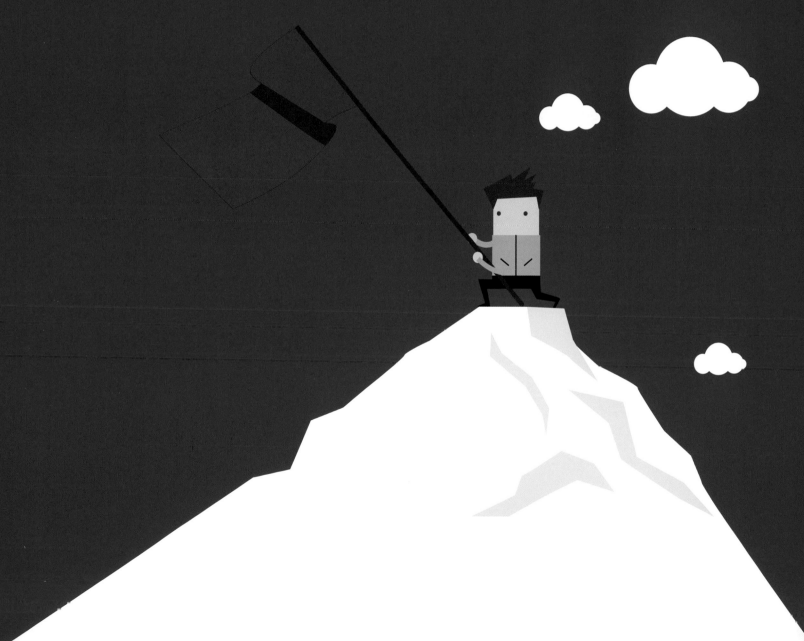

10**Ten**

Make 10 ten-year goals

Purpose

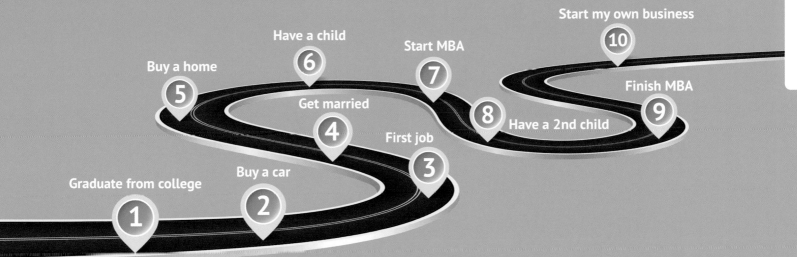

Start my own business

10

Have a child

6

Start MBA

7

Finish MBA

9

Buy a home

5

Get married

4

Have a 2nd child

8

First job

3

Buy a car

2

Graduate from college

1

The 10 Ten Challenge invites you to make 10 ten-year goals. Think about where you would like to be in 10 years. Where will you be in your profession? Where will you be in your family life? Where will you be financially? Write down at least 10 ten-year goals and put them somewhere you can see them periodically or even daily.

Lewis Carroll, who penned *Alice in Wonderland*, said, "If you don't know where you are going, any road will get you there." Your short list of 10 goals will define where you want to go and will help you choose which road to take daily. Your goals will give you direction and purpose when you face rough times and will inspire you to go beyond what you would normally do when times are good. It will be interesting to see how many of your goals you actually accomplish and where your quest takes you!

Purpose

Social

GiftList

Ask 10 people what you're good at

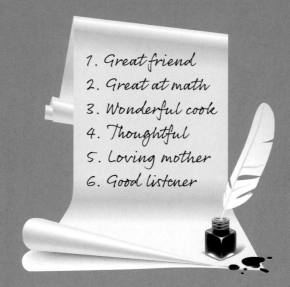

1. Great friend
2. Great at math
3. Wonderful cook
4. Thoughtful
5. Loving mother
6. Good listener

The Gift List Challenge invites you to compile a list of your talents or gifts by asking 10 people what they think you're good at and then put their responses into a single list. It's that simple. Don't be shy. Your friends and family will be more than willing to help you out. Ask them to send you an email or write down their answers as they dictate them to you on the spot.

Discovering your strengths can be empowering! Sometimes we fall into the trap of comparing our imperfections with others' strengths. The reality is that we all have a long list of strengths—the list is just different for each of us. When you see your gift list, you will be positively overwhelmed with how good you actually are. Armed with an understanding of your strengths, you will be able to better focus your energy in everything you do—for your career, hobbies, and social interactions. Get ready to discover a long list of talents and gifts you didn't even realize you had!

GreatDay

Say it's going to be a great day

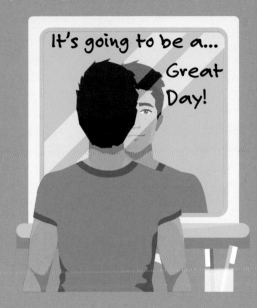

The Great Day Challenge invites you to say out loud, "It's going to be a great day!" once a day for the next 30 days, preferably first thing in the morning. Stop reading right now and try this out loud. The immediate feeling of exhilaration and hope it creates is amazing. The act of proclaiming aloud such a positive statement is quite powerful.

You've heard it said that you are the master of your own destiny, so it shouldn't be that hard to be the master of a single day. You control whether or not it's going to be a good day, not the forces of the universe acting upon you. Yes, things will happen to you (good and bad), but you are the one who determines how you will respond. Believe that the day will be great from the start, and it will. Have a great day!

Look**Forward**

Write about an anticipated event

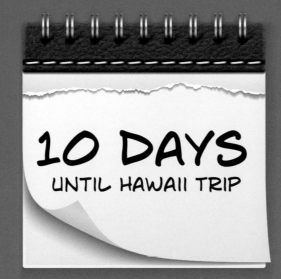

The Look Forward Challenge invites you to write down one thought a day about an anticipated event for the next 30 days. The event can be as simple as going to see a new movie when it's released or perhaps an upcoming vacation or friend's wedding. It just needs to be something that's going to happen 30 days or more from today. Write down your thoughts in your journal or on your computer. Your daily entry can be about anything you are anticipating—from the food you will eat to the sites you will visit to the people you will see. If you miss a day, just write two thoughts the next day.

Interestingly enough, anticipating an event can often be more satisfying than the event itself. When you look forward to an activity, it brings a sense of excitement and happiness into your being—brightening your outlook and creating hope for the future. This enhanced perspective makes the challenges of life easier to hurdle. Pondering or visualizing an activity in advance also helps you more fully experience the actual event. What are you looking forward to?

Me**Remembered**

Write your obituary

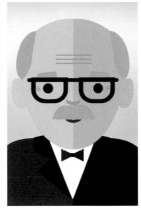

JOHN DOE, 1975-2058

The Me Remembered Challenge invites you to write your own obituary. While at first this might seem morbid, instead, think of it as a way to consider your end goals. Ask yourself: "When I die, how would I like to be remembered? What would I like others to say about me? What are the things that are most important to me? What things do I want to accomplish?" Obituaries are short and concise, so make your words count.

Writing your own obituary is an interesting way to ponder the purpose of your life. As you do so, this clarified purpose may help you refocus your energies on the things that matter most to you. It may help you to become more aware and considerate of the people around you. It may help you to quicken your pace to ensure you accomplish all that you want to do. Whatever the outcome, pondering your purpose is a positive exercise that can make your life more satisfying now and in the future.

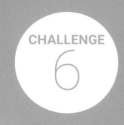

Mission**Possible**

Write a personal mission statement

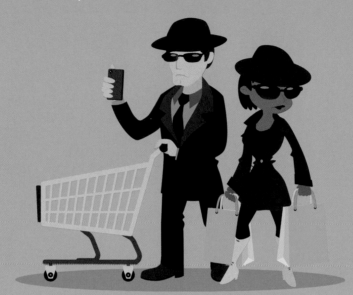

The Mission Possible Challenge invites you to write a personal mission statement. This is much more than a catchy slogan. A mission statement will clearly express what drives you and what is important to you. It will help you define your direction and purpose in life. It will be the foundation for your goals and will help you evaluate whether or not you are living true to your self-defined purpose. Stephen R. Covey, author of *The 7 Habits of Highly Effective People,* wrote that a mission statement is "like a personal constitution, the basis for making major, life-directing decisions, the basis for making daily decisions."

Set aside some time to think about what you'd like your mission statement to be. Write your ideas on paper or on a private online journal. What are you passionate about? What brings you joy? What are you naturally good at? What do you stand for? Which ethics and values are important to you? How would you like to influence others? Contemplate these answers as you create a purposeful statement that captures the essence of who you are. Don't worry about making it perfect. Start with a rough draft and you can change it over time.

RememberMe

Spend 300 minutes writing a memoir

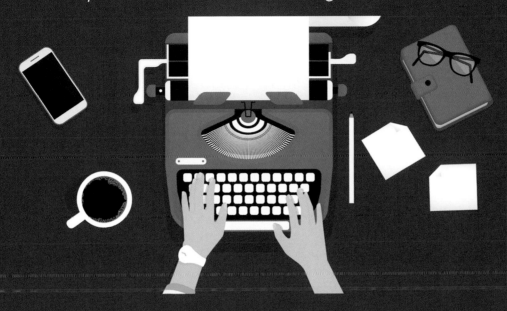

The Remember Me Challenge invites you to spend 300 minutes over the next 30 days writing an autobiography. Get a notebook, set up a blog, or keep a document on your computer. It's easier if you plan a set time each day, or you could "binge write" on certain evenings or weekends. Start with your earliest memories or write about your most recent experiences first. You can always make changes as you go, so don't worry about making it perfect.

Writing about your life is therapeutic. It can help you understand how you've become the person you are, and give insight as to who you still hope to become. You'll also recognize all the people who have been instrumental in your life. A memoir is one of the biggest gifts you can give your posterity. They will learn your history first-hand, gaining insight into the details of your life and what you learned along the way. There's no better time than the present. Get started while your experiences are still fresh in your memory. It will be easier than you think!

PriorityPlan

Set personal goals

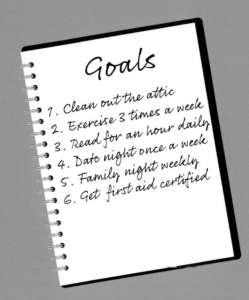

Goals
1. Clean out the attic
2. Exercise 3 times a week
3. Read for an hour daily
4. Date night once a week
5. Family night weekly
6. Get first aid certified

Purpose

Emotional

Social

Physical

Occupational

Financial

The Priority Plan Challenge invites you to set personal goals for the upcoming year. Many people do this in January, but you can do it any time of the year. Consider setting goals for each area of your life: personal, family, work, health, mental, social, etc. Don't go overboard—choose realistic, achievable goals. Create goals that are measurable so it will be clear when you've achieved them. As you complete each goal, record it where you can keep track of them, like in your planner or on your desk.

Setting specific personal goals will help you focus your energy and time to accomplish what is most important and will bring definition and purpose to your life. Writing them down will greatly increase the chance they will happen. When you actually accomplish your goals, you will have greater confidence and personal satisfaction that may propel you to even higher levels. So, what are your goals?

TrueNorth

Ponder your purpose

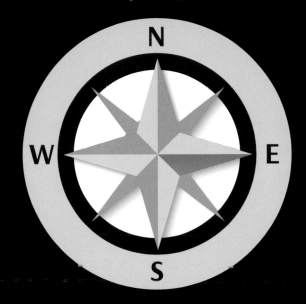

The True North Challenge invites you to spend a few minutes each day for the next 30 days thinking about your purpose in life. The challenge is easy. Simply ponder your personal mission statement each day, thinking about how you can apply the principles to the situations you are facing in life. If you don't have a personal mission statement, then start by doing the Mission Possible Challenge: contemplate the purpose of your life and craft a simple statement that encapsulates it. You can determine when you will ponder your purpose and how long you will do it each day.

Finding and embracing your purpose can make a tremendous impact on what you are able to accomplish as you go through life. You will define success for your life, most likely in a way that is very different from how the world defines it. As you face the challenges and influences of the world around you, you will stay true to your true north. Don't worry that you might not live up to your expectations. Thinking about your purpose in life will help you get there eventually, as you continue to face your true north.

CHALLENGE 10

Emotional

40Day
Give up something for 40 days

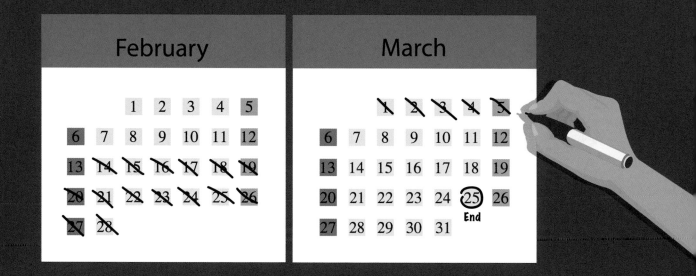

The 40 Day Challenge invites you to give up something for 40 out of the next 45 days—you get five exception days. The best part of this challenge is that you get to pick what you will give up. Choose something that is meaningful to you, something you may want to cut back on long term, or even cease entirely.

Too often our bodies control our spirits and minds. Hunger, fatigue, emotions, and cravings lead us to indulge in things that may not be good for us. Turn this tendency around and gain control of your body! Choose something you know you can give up successfully, even if it seems like a tiny change. Small habit changes can springboard a process of shifting other patterns in our lives, leading to better health and greater happiness. It is empowering to be in control and realize your capability to accomplish great things!

100**Thanks**
Say "thank you" 100 times

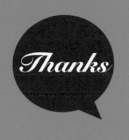

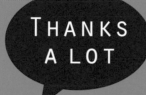

Thanks

Thank you

Thanks so much

THANKS
A LOT

Thank you
very much

Emotional

Social

The 100 Thanks Challenge invites you to say "thank you" 100 times over the next 30 days (about 3 times/day). The goal of this challenge is to train your mind to look for things that you are thankful for, ultimately becoming aware of all the good in your life. As you begin to regularly thank people, your mindset will change. Things that might normally irritate you will become less so—ultimately making you a happier person. In the process, people around you will be happier, too!

Every time you interact with others, you have the opportunity to express appreciation. Seize that moment! When you notice someone doing something kind or generous—whether for you or another person—express your gratitude. Think about those who affect your life; be sure to thank them as well. Thank your neighbors, your family, your children's teachers, and even people you encounter while running your errands or shopping. Showing gratitude strengthens relationships, helps us make new friends, and improves both our mental and physical health. By the way, thanks for giving this challenge a try!

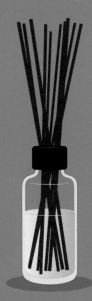

Aroma Therapy

15 aromatherapy sessions

Emotional

Physical

The Aroma Therapy Challenge invites you to use aromatherapy 15 times in the next 30 days to help you relax. Aromatherapy is the practice of inhaling the aroma of natural oils extracted from various plants, which can benefit both the body and the mind. It sounds more complicated than it is. All you need is an essential oil that promotes relaxation like lavender, bergamot, jasmine, chamomile, peppermint, or sandalwood. The easiest way to find essential oils is online, but many stores carry them, too. For a more personal scent, you can even make your own blend of calming oils.

Some ways to enjoy aromatherapy are: (1) put a few drops on a cotton ball, (2) add a few drops to a cup of steaming hot water, (3) use in a diffuser, (4) put several drops in your bath, or (5) dilute a few drops in a teaspoon of olive oil or coconut oil and massage into the skin. Aromatherapy is a nice, relaxing break during the day, or it can soothe and relax the body at bedtime. Combine aromatherapy with deep breathing or meditation for increased calming effects. Aromatherapy is a simple pleasure of life—see what it can do for you.

Double**Dare**

Try 2 new things

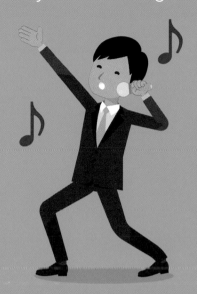

The Double Dare Challenge invites you to try two new things during the next 30 days. Try a new food, like octopus. Go to the opera. Volunteer at a shelter. Go rock climbing. Change your hairstyle. Write a letter to your senator. Sing at an open mic night. There are so many options. What will you choose? Make it something that is personally challenging. The more you put yourself out there, the more meaningful and memorable the experience will be.

Trying new things forces you to grow and expand your interests. It's difficult to break out of familiar routines, but this can be an opportunity to meet new people or increase your passion about one of your current interests. This challenge will give you the opportunity to try something new, build self-confidence, open your mind, and fuel creativity. Perhaps you will overcome a fear, participate more in your community, or find a new hobby to enjoy. Trying something new can be intimidating, but you just might find something you really like that you never knew about!

CHALLENGE
14

Emotional

ExcuseMe

No negative self-talk

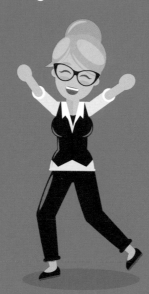

The Excuse Me Challenge invites you to not say anything negative about yourself for 30 days. If you catch yourself doing that, quickly say something positive about yourself and go forward from there. On the surface, the challenge may seem easy, but unfortunately negative self-talk is a habit for many. People make self-deprecating comments as a form of humor or in an effort to be modest or humble, but such comments are not good at all.

How you think and speak of yourself can have a huge impact on how you actually perform. Think of what would happen if you constantly pointed out your friend or associate's weaknesses—they would feel awful and might give up on trying to do better. If you point out another's strengths instead, it would have a tremendous effect on how they feel and how they live their life. Be kind to yourself, just like you would be kind to a friend. Speak positively about yourself and you will become the most positive version of yourself.

FlowerPower

Keep flowers on your table

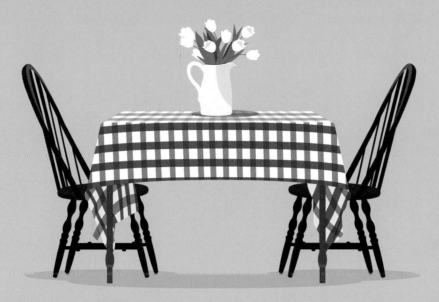

The Flower Power Challenge invites you to beautify your surroundings by keeping fresh flowers on your table at home or your desk at work for 30 days. You'll need to replace them each week with new flowers (ideally at the start of the work week) so that you can continually feel the energy and peace that nature brings. Start by picking up flowers from a local florist, grocery store, or even from your backyard. Depending on the type of flowers you choose, the cost can be surprisingly reasonable.

Flowers can actually boost your mood, reduce stress, and improve concentration. They can also combat depression and anxiety and can make your day seem more enjoyable. A beautiful floral arrangement in your home or workplace can generate improvements in productivity, creativity, and problem solving. Always stop and smell the flowers. Enjoy their beauty and see what flowers do for you!

Good**Culture**

Visit a museum

Emotional

Social

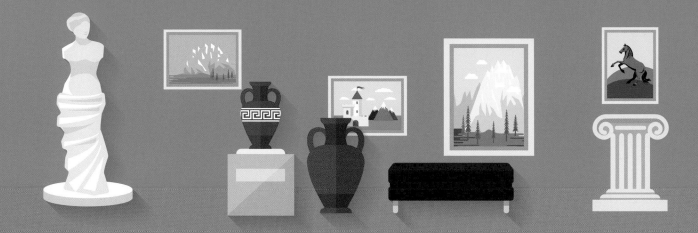

The Good Culture Challenge invites you to visit a museum. Any type of museum will do, including: art, science, sports, technology, or even a wax museum! Check your nearby museums for any traveling exhibits, like the *Titanic* disaster or ancient Egyptian relics. Contact the museum about its hours and any discounts it has available. Many public libraries offer museum passports that get you in for free or at heavily discounted rates. Invite a friend and make it a fun occasion.

Museums provide real, hands-on learning experiences. You can wander at your own pace, perusing and soaking in what you want and walking past whatever doesn't peak your interest. Museums can broaden your perspective of the world, letting you experience artifacts from distant lands, different times, and diverse cultures. Visit a museum and expand your horizons.

Good**Reception**

No television

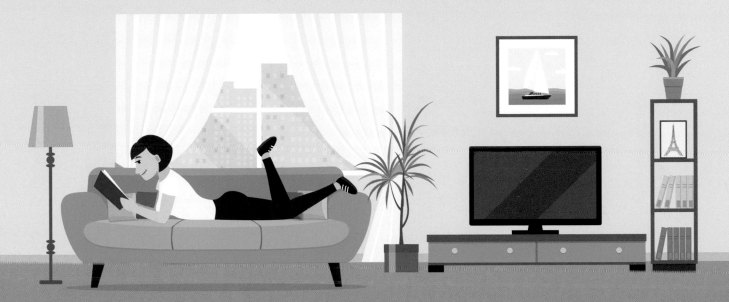

Emotional

The Good Reception Challenge invites you to limit TV watching and instead tune into yourself for the next 30 days. For the full experience, turn off your TV for 30 consecutive days. If that's too extreme for you, limit your TV viewing to a single program, a certain length of time, or only on weekends. Remember, this is a challenge! You'll find plenty of free time on your hands—fill it with something you've wanted to do for a long time.

Excessive TV watching can lead to obesity, social exclusion, and sleeping difficulties. Similar to drug addiction, TV provides an escape from reality to enjoy a fantasy world that's free from problems. Letting go of this TV "fix" may not be easy at first, but once you find something valuable to do in its place, you'll wonder why you ever spent so much time watching TV before!

Great**Start**

Make your bed

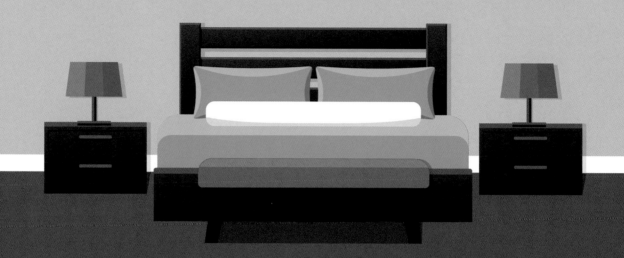

The Great Start Challenge invites you to begin your day with a success—making your bed—for 25 out of the next 30 days. There's no need to go crazy and achieve military bed-making standards. Fluff your pillows, pull up your sheets and bedspread, and tuck in any loose ends. You can make your bed in less than 60 seconds. If you wake up earlier than your sleeping partner, you can still gently straighten your side of the bed without any disruption.

Making your bed in the morning establishes a pattern of productivity and order that will transcend into other parts of your life. Order begets order, and success breeds success. Even though making your bed may seem pointless—since you're just going to get back in and mess it up later on—the impact to your life can be powerful and positive! Give yourself the gift of success each morning, as well as a tidy and more peaceful home environment to return to at the end of each day.

Green Thumb

Grow a plant or garden

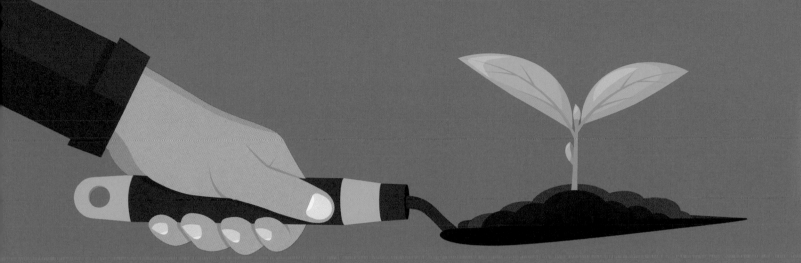

The Green Thumb Challenge invites you to grow a plant or garden. You can grow one that is large or small, outdoors or indoors, in the ground or in a pot, edible or simply decorative. You can even buy a plant that's already potted and keep it on your desk. If gardening is new to you, ask a friend or family member for help. Gardening is pretty simple—you'll catch on quickly and will enjoy the process.

Gardening is healthy for the body and soothing for the soul. It is satisfying to see the results of your labor as the plants grow and develop, reconnecting you with Mother Earth. Gardening can give you a healthy dose of vitamin D, as well as positively affect your strength, dexterity, endurance, problem solving, sensory awareness, and learning abilities. Give gardening a try and see how it grows on you!

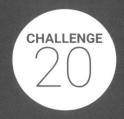

I'mOkay
List 30 good things about yourself

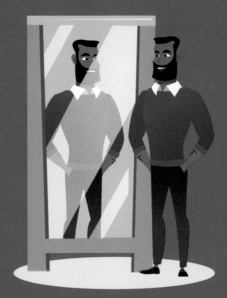

The I'm Okay Challenge invites you to give a compliment to the one who deserves it the most—yourself! You are your biggest critic; it's time to reverse that pattern and send yourself positive messages instead. For the next 30 days, write down one good thing about yourself every day. Keep your list on your desk, in your planner, or on your computer desktop—somewhere easily visible so it can lift your spirits throughout the day.

As you shift from negative self-talk and start to embrace what is truly great about you, your doubts, fears, and discouraging thoughts will diminish. As you discover your strengths, you will expand your potential. A good self-image will give you confidence when expressing your opinion. The better we treat ourselves, the better we will treat others around us, creating a ripple effect of positivity in the world.

LuckyDuck

List 30 fortunate events

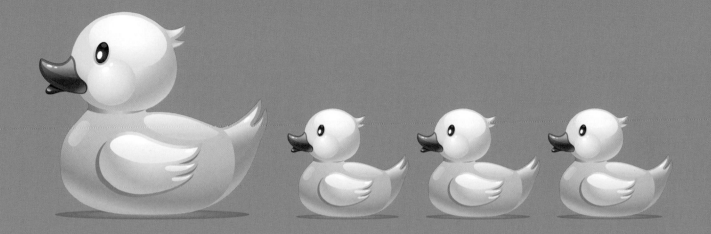

The Lucky Duck Challenge invites you to recognize how lucky you are by listing one fortunate thing that happens to you each day for 30 days. Identify something that shows how you were in the right place at the right time. Big or small—anything positive qualifies. Perhaps you got a green light when you needed it, the checkout line was empty at the store, you were able to leave work early, or you ran into an old friend. If you miss one day, then look for two things the next day. Write your lucky events in your journal or log them on your phone. It's a wonderful thing to remind yourself how very fortunate you are.

As we focus on the positive, the negative fades into the background or goes completely unnoticed—making your life much more enjoyable. Here's the crazy part: your life can actually change for the better. Positive thoughts breed positive outcomes. When we believe that positive things happen to us, more and more positive things actually do happen to us. This may sound far-fetched, but try your luck and see.

CHALLENGE
22

Emotional

LOL
Laugh out loud daily

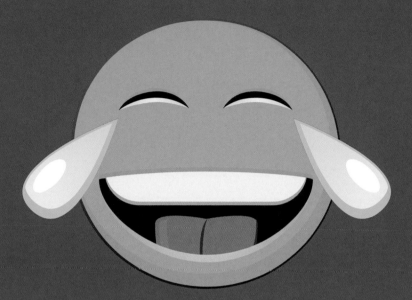

The LOL Challenge invites you to literally laugh out loud at least once a day for the next 30 days. If you miss a day, laugh more the next day. You're probably thinking this is silly and that you can't make yourself laugh. You're right, but you can place yourself in an environment that promotes laughter. Listen to a funny morning show on the radio. Hang out with a friend who always makes you laugh. Watch your favorite sitcom or a funny video on the Internet. Spend time with children. It will be easier than you think.

Laughing is truly medicine for the soul and body. It reduces stress hormones, boosts your immune system, lowers blood pressure, relieves pain, and makes you feel better. Laughter even improves memory and increases creativity. Laughter isn't such a silly thing after all. Experience the benefits of laughter every day because, as Andrew Carnegie said, "There is little success where there is little laughter."

Lost**Baggage**
Forgive 5 people

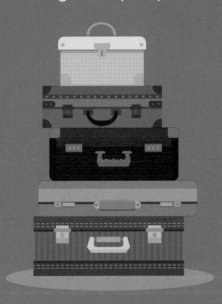

The Lost Baggage Challenge invites you to forgive five people in the next 30 days. On a piece of paper, make a list of five people and briefly list what they did that harmed or bothered you. Next, destroy the piece of paper. That's right...rip it up, shred it, let it go! If the offense crosses your mind later on, don't dwell on it—let the thought pass. There's no need to talk to the person, unless you feel it would be helpful. Your list may range from people who did a little annoying thing to something awful that greatly affected your life. If your list is longer than five items, write those down too—the challenge will be even more impactful!

Harboring bad or hurtful feelings can be troubling, stressful, and detrimental to your health. Forgiveness literally lifts burdens from your body—decreasing physical and emotional pain, lowering heart rate and blood pressure, and reducing the level of cortisol, the stress hormone. Forgiving may seem impossible to do in some cases. Just strive to let go as best you can and free yourself from that burdensome weight.

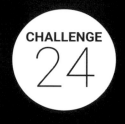
Mouth**Wash**

No swearing

Emotional

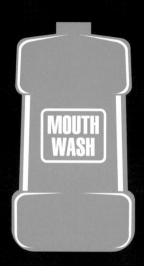

The Mouth Wash Challenge invites you to not use any swear words for the next 30 days. If you slip up, just restate your sentence without the swear word and call it good. For an added challenge, try to not use any substitute swear words either. The real challenge here may be expanding your vocabulary to find more appropriate words to replace the swear words. It's actually an excellent exercise for your mind to find new ways of expressing yourself.

At first glance, removing swear words from your vocabulary might seem like a pointless exercise. After all, the shock value of swear words can bring added impact to your communications. Stop and think though. Will your associates respect you more or less if you stop using swear words? Exercising restraint and being courteous to those around you are noble attributes. This is a hard habit to break. If you don't succeed right away, just keep trying—it will get easier!

My**Word**

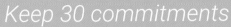
Keep 30 commitments

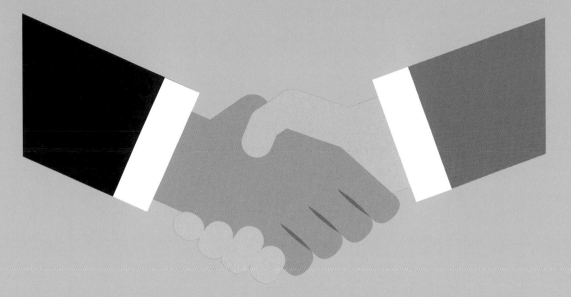

The My Word Challenge invites you to follow through on 30 promises you make to yourself in the next 30 days. Each morning, think of one thing you want to do that day and promise yourself that you'll do it. Then do it! It's that simple. If you don't follow through for some reason, do it the next day or commit to do two new things the following day. The goal of this challenge is not to make big commitments—it's to *keep* your commitments. So be realistic and keep your plans simple.

We all like to think of ourselves as trustworthy. When we make a promise to another person, we don't want to let them down. Yet, most of us break commitments with ourselves far too often—and if we break commitments with ourselves, can we really be trusted? This challenge may be truly transformational. It will help you stop making commitments that you aren't going to keep, and only make those that you will keep. Conquer this challenge and become someone with integrity whom everyone can truly trust.

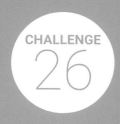

Pablo**Picasso**

Paint a picture

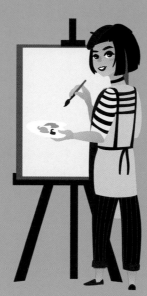

The Pablo Picasso Challenge invites you to paint a picture. Paint with watercolors, acrylics, oil paint, or even finger paint. Paint on a canvas board, art paper, clothing, a piece of wood, or paint a mural on your wall. Paint with a brush or any tool you can think of, like a sponge, spray gun, stick, or your hand. Your painting can be as abstract or realistic as you'd like. Just paint something and enjoy the process.

Painting is something children love to do at school, yet adults don't often think to do it. Besides being fun, painting can also be therapeutic and a wonderful way to communicate in a different kind of language. It stimulates both sides of the brain, allowing logic and creativity to work together, also letting the heart express emotion without even realizing it. Painting can be a relaxing escape from our day-to-day lives. Get those paints ready and see what appears!

Re**Route**

Take 10 different routes to work

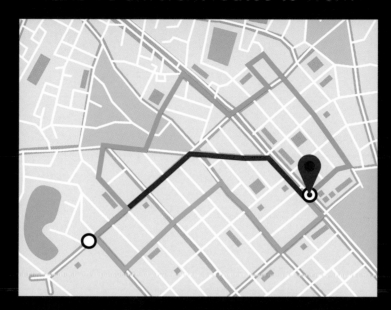

The Re Route Challenge invites you to take 10 different routes to work in the next 30 days. The purpose of taking different routes is to stimulate your mind by introducing the unexpected to your day. You can plan out the route changes in advance or do them spontaneously. Be sure to leave home earlier to allow for any timing differences. If your commute doesn't allow for many route changes, look for simple ways to alter how you walk out of your home, from your car, through the train station, or even through your building to get to your office—maybe even switch your mode of transportation to mix things up.

In life, we often fall into ruts, repeating the same old routine again and again. In fact, that's the way our brain likes it—because it knows what to expect and doesn't need to work as hard. By introducing variety and spontaneity into our lives, we put our brain to work, keeping our minds sharp and making our lives interesting! Be an overachiever and look for other ways to keep your life fresh: work from a different location, try a new lunch place, taste a new food, meet someone new, or simply change your computer background. Keeping it fresh is fun and healthy.

Reader's **Dozen**

Read 13 books

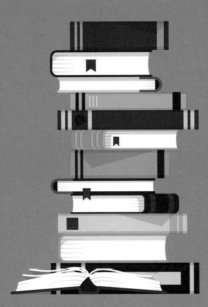

The Reader's Dozen Challenge invites you to read 13 books in one year. The books can be fiction or nonfiction and can be any genre: romance, mystery, science, religion, business—whatever grabs your interest. It doesn't matter how long the book is. If you are having a hard time coming up with ideas, ask a friend for recommendations or peruse the various lists of best-sellers in your newspaper or online. You could also join a book club, allowing you to meet new people as an added benefit.

Reading books offers the obvious benefits of entertainment, gaining knowledge, expanding your vocabulary, and stimulating your brain. Added bonuses to reading books include improving your memory, giving you a greater ability to focus, reducing stress in your life, and preventing or slowing degenerative brain disease. Which book are you most excited to read first?

RealWorld

No social media

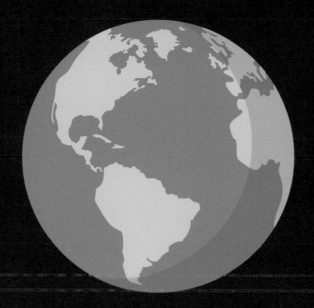

The Real World Challenge invites you to take a break from social media for 30 days. That's right, no Facebook, Snapchat, Twitter, and the like for 30 days—a real challenge! Texts and email are still fine during the challenge, as well as LinkedIn, since it's often work related. The easiest way to avoid social media is to remove the apps from your devices so they won't be a temptation. If you're worried about your friends thinking you're rude for not replying, announce your challenge before you sign off of social media. Invite your friends to do the same!

We have become so intensely addicted to social media that we waste incredible amounts of time that could be better spent on things that really matter. Countless times each day, we grab our phones and feel an unconscious rush when we see something we like. We can easily get caught up scrolling mindlessly or commenting on things that don't matter. Perhaps even worse, social media causes us to compare ourselves with the seemingly perfect lives of others, leaving us feeling inadequate and left out. Ironically, social media actually causes us to withdraw from those around us. Give yourself a break from unreality and plug into the real world instead!

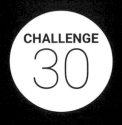

CHALLENGE
30

ScaredyCat

Face one fear

Emotional

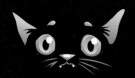

The Scaredy Cat Challenge invites you to face one fear. If your heart rate went up a bit just thinking about facing a fear, you're not alone. Our fears are real, they are physical, and they can seem impossible to tackle. Don't worry—it doesn't have to stay that way. Whether you have a fear of heights, public speaking, or even being near spiders, facing that fear head on or gradually and repeatedly exposing yourself to triggers surrounding your fear will actually change your life.

Some fears can actually be disabling, holding you back from getting more out of life or even just getting through normal daily tasks. Even if the fear seems inconsequential, like being afraid of snakes, facing that fear will be empowering, giving you more confidence in yourself and your ability to overcome obstacles. This challenge only asks you to face one fear, so brace yourself. You can totally do this!

TreeHugger

Enjoy nature for 300 minutes

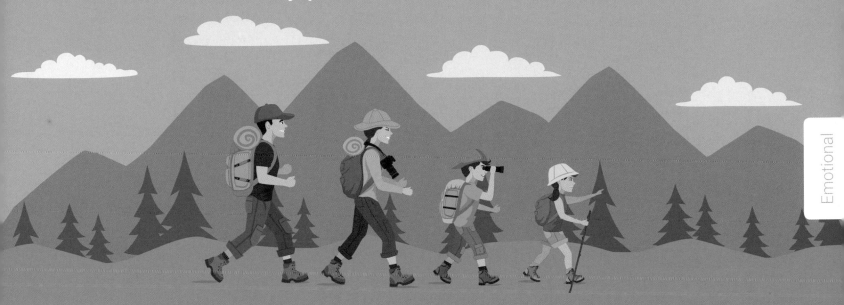

Emotional

The Tree Hugger Challenge invites you to enjoy nature for 300 minutes over the next 30 days— about 10 minutes per day. Choose something you enjoy doing. Enjoy lunch on a park bench or take a hike on a walking trail. Go fishing, boating, camping, or to the beach. You can get your 300 minutes in all in one day or spread it out over the next 30 days. Both options have their advantages.

Being in nature is therapeutic. It reduces stress, improves mental health, and increases mindfulness. Even a few minutes of sitting with nature transitions your mind into a relaxed state, which reduces blood pressure. In our busy lives, we can become disconnected from the beauty of the natural world. Reconnecting with nature can help us reconnect with ourselves, and help us to remember who we are and what's really important to us, easing feelings of isolation and anxiety. Being in nature also reminds us that we're not just individuals—we're a part of a larger, beautiful world.

William**Shakespeare**

Write a poem

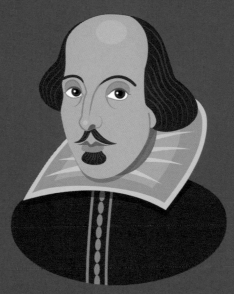

The William Shakespeare Challenge invites you to write a poem. Initially, you might think that you can't write poetry—but you can. If you're not sure what to write about, describe a person in your life, something you love, a recent experience, or express an emotion that has been bubbling to the surface. Poetry is like painting a picture with words. You can use any style that suits you and make the poem any length you'd like. There are no rules, just write.

Want to get smarter? Write a poem. Writing poetry improves cognitive function as you expand your vocabulary, think out meter and rhythm, and find creative ways to articulate your thoughts and feelings. The process of writing your poem can release and heal deep emotions, which can be therapeutic for you and beneficial to those who read it. You can do it! Take the challenge, enjoy the process, and get in touch with your Shakespearean side!

Be**Friend**

Do 12 things with a friend

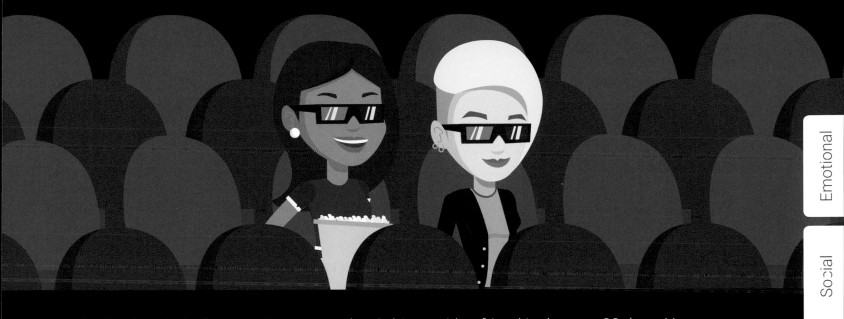

Emotional

Social

The Be Friend Challenge invites you to do 12 things with a friend in the next 30 days. You can choose whether you'd like to do all 12 with one friend or split the experiences among several friends. You can even do the same activity 12 times this month—as long as it's with a friend. Eat out, go for a walk, help your friend with a project, or drop by to visit. Be creative! Just try to pick something that gives you some time to talk with each other or share an experience together so you can strengthen your bond.

Sometimes we get so busy with work and family that we forget to make time for friends. As children, it was natural for us to want to spend time with friends, but it's just as important for us now as adults. If you are new to your area and don't have friends nearby, get out and make some new friends. Try inviting other folks over who are also new to the area; they need to make new friends too! If you have plenty of friends already, get together more often. Invest time in your friendships and they will last you a lifetime.

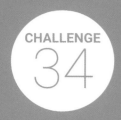

CHALLENGE
34

Be**There**

Put your cell phone away

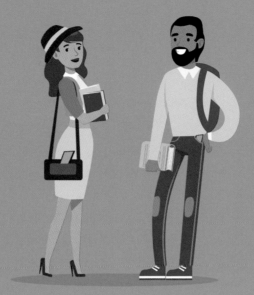

Social

The Be There Challenge invites you to put your cell phone away when you're with other people for 30 days. The idea is to focus on people when you're with people—your cell phone can wait. Not only is it rude to ignore your company, you are missing out on one of the most enjoyable parts of life—interpersonal relationships. If your conversation slows down, be the one to liven it up or simply enjoy being there, sharing that moment without words. Give others your full attention and be present!

Smartphones have become an addiction. We impulsively grab for our phones with each alert or notification, anxious to find out what important information just came in. When we're bored, we look to our phones in hopes of being entertained. Like any addiction, it's not healthy—but being present with other people is good for you, in fact, it's vital for your health. It's not as hard as it seems. Power off your phone and power on the life around you!

Come**Together**

Join a group

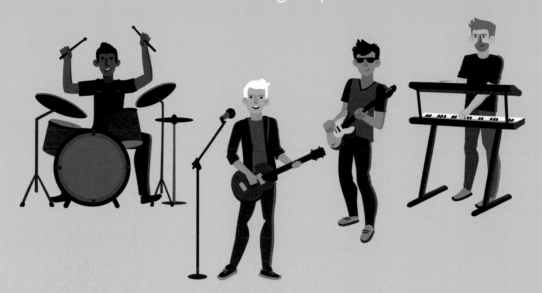

The Come Together Challenge invites you to join a group or a club and attend at least one meeting. It can be any kind of group—a book club, a band, a sports team, a church choir, a volunteer organization, or even one that goes biking every weekend. Find a group that interests you. If you can't find the type of group you're looking for, start your own!

Meeting up with others who love what you're interested in is fun and rewarding. Together you can accomplish much more than you'd be able to do on your own. Joining a group allows you to help and motivate each other, and hold each other accountable. Collaborating also gives you an opportunity to grow your own ideas or help others grow theirs. Being in a group setting lets you practice patience, selflessness, and the ability to resolve conflicts—all great life skills. As you spend time together, you will bond, feel valued, and find a greater sense of identity. Come together, right now!

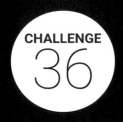

Family Tree

Talk with 7 relatives

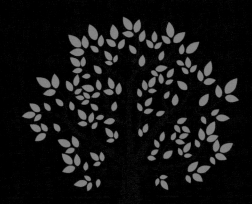

The Family Tree Challenge invites you to reach out to seven relatives and have a conversation with each one over the next 30 days. You can reach out to immediate family or distant relatives, but you should choose people that you don't normally talk to on a day-to-day basis. A phone conversation is fine, but if you can visit in person that's even better. The length and detail of the conversations are up to you and can vary depending on who you are talking with.

There really is nothing like family. Family ties can be some of the strongest ties you will have in life. There's a built-in trust factor and connection with relatives that allows you to talk about subjects you wouldn't normally feel comfortable talking about. Family can give you help you wouldn't normally get—or be willing to accept—from friends. Especially intriguing is the fact that as you understand your family better, you are able to better understand yourself. Be there for your family and they will be there for you!

GreatJob

Write 10 LinkedIn recommendations

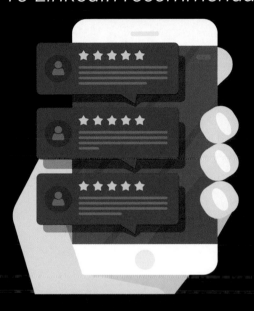

The Great Job Challenge invites you to write 10 LinkedIn recommendations over the next 30 days. Browse your LinkedIn contacts for people you feel positively about and write a recommendation for 10 of them. Grab the reader's attention with your first sentence, explain your relationship to the person, mention specifically why you respect that person, use examples to make your recommendation powerful, and end with a short, solid statement of endorsement. Before your recommendation posts to their profile, your contact will get a chance to review it.

Your contacts will be delighted when they receive your recommendation! It will likely make their day. Some may reciprocate by writing a recommendation for you—but that's not the goal here. The goal is to do something nice for someone else and to practice focusing on the good in others. As you move more toward an outward focus, life will become more enjoyable. Take a few minutes and make someone's day!

HeartFelt

Tell 20 people why you appreciate them

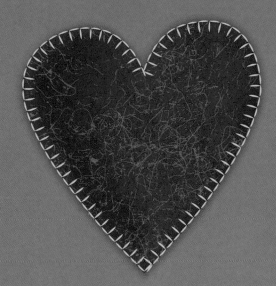

The Heart Felt Challenge invites you to tell 20 different people why you appreciate them over the next 30 days. This is actually harder than it sounds. First you need to reflect on why you appreciate someone, then you need to actually tell that person—which may feel a bit awkward. What may be difficult in this challenge is finding 20 different people, stepping out of your comfort zone, and expressing appreciation for people you might not know or talk to that frequently.

We often show that we appreciate people through our actions: by helping, listening, or smiling. However, if you truly appreciate someone, it's important to tell them too—even if it doesn't come naturally. The more we express appreciation for others, the more we will actually appreciate them. Furthermore, the more we feel connected and appreciated, the happier and healthier we become. What do you have to lose? Contemplate those you appreciate in your life, speak up, and let them know.

HelpMe

Ask 5 people for help

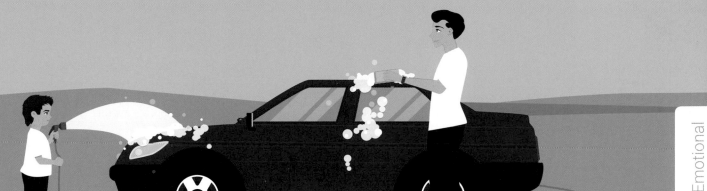

Emotional

Social

The Help Me Challenge invites you to ask five people for help in the next 30 days. Most people are comfortable offering help to others, but are very uncomfortable asking for help from others. Perhaps it is pride. Perhaps it just feels awkward. Whatever the cause, when we refuse to ask for help, we are missing out. Receiving help may enable us to do something we wouldn't be able to do otherwise. More importantly, by accepting help from others, we allow others to experience the joy of serving. Ask for help and make someone's day!

It may take some work to get out of the "I can do it myself" mindset and start asking for help. Think of things that you could do yourself but could still benefit from others' help. Ask for feedback on a presentation you are preparing. Ask a friend to come by and give you ideas on how to decorate or landscape. Think of ways others could make your life easier. Ask a friend to carpool. Invite someone to help you plan a party or do a big project. Ask for advice about a problem you're having. People love to help. By asking for help you will actually be helping others fulfill this inherent human need.

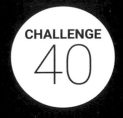

HighsNLows

Discuss your day as a family

Emotional

Social

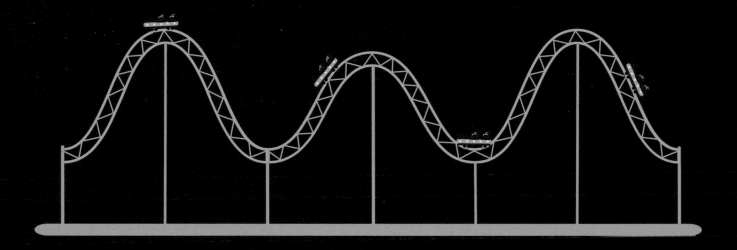

The Highs N Lows Challenge invites you to discuss your day as a family for 20 out of the next 30 days. Here's how it works: Each person takes a turn sharing the best thing (their "high") and the worst thing (their "low") that happened that day. If dinnertime is not practical for your family, pick another, like bedtime. If you don't live with family, try it with your roommates or set a time to phone a friend. Talking about the triumphs and trials of life can be fun, relaxing, and even therapeutic.

Just like food is fuel for our bodies, talking in person is fuel for our brains and sustenance for our hearts. In our world of social media and texting, it's especially important to make time to interact face to face. As we share the ups and downs of life, we build relationships, learn from each other, and create stronger bonds. Everyone will benefit as you solve problems together and support one another. Give it a try—this may end up being your new high point of the day!

ImprovNight

Play improv games

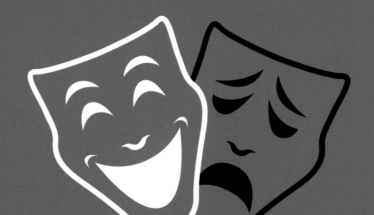

Social

Physical

The Improv Night Challenge invites you to participate in improv (improvisation) games. If you've never tried improv, get ready to laugh, have fun, and enjoy a challenge for your brain. If you can't find an improv event to attend, then you can plan your own improv night. There are tons of improv game ideas available online. The basic format is to gather several people together, then divide into two or more teams of 3–5 each. Ask someone who's experienced with improv to be the referee or host of the games.

The idea behind improv is to improvise or make up things as you go. Not only is this hilarious, it is also a great brain activity. Your brain is a pattern recognition machine. As soon as it recognizes a pattern, it goes into "sleep mode" and lets a preset, automatic response take over. Since improv is totally random, the brain is hard at work the whole time—building your creativity and your ability to think on your feet. Get your friends to try it with you. It could become your new favorite night out!

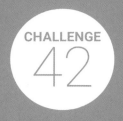

CHALLENGE
42

Keep**Warm**
Donate an old coat

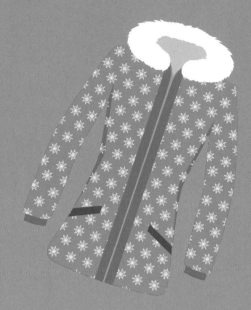

Emotional

Social

The Keep Warm Challenge invites you to donate a new or used winter coat to someone in need. The coat can be of any size or style. You can give the coat directly to someone you know who would appreciate it or donate it to a local homeless shelter or thrift store. While you're at it, consider donating other items that you no longer need and maybe even donate some cash. Completing this challenge is simple though, as you only need to donate one used coat.

Giving is a great way to shift the focus from yourself to others, resulting in greater personal happiness—one of life's pleasing paradoxes. In fact, people who are generally happier are in overall better health and have increased life expectancy. It's also nice to think about how you give to those in need because you can, and because it's the right thing to do. Help someone else keep warm and warm your heart at the same time.

Litter Bug

Keep your neighborhood clean

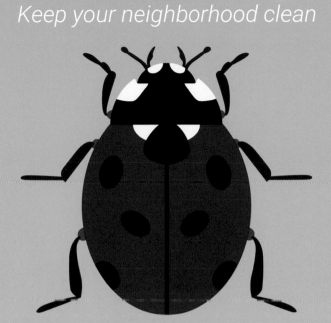

Emotional

Social

Physical

The Litter Bug Challenge invites you to make the world a cleaner place by picking up one piece of trash for 21 out of the next 30 days. You can pick up more trash each day if you want to, but you only need to pick up one item to get credit for the day. The goal is to make it a habit, not just a one-time major cleanup day. Pick up trash that has blown into your yard—before it blows into someone else's yard! Bring a bag to collect trash when you walk in your neighborhood. Pick up something in the parking lot as you head into work or a store. Every little bit makes a difference.

In addition to the obvious benefits of making your surroundings nicer for yourself and for others, this habit can help you in other ways. As you search for trash to pick up, it will help you focus on what you can do for the world instead of what the world can do for you. This mindset makes life easier to traverse and can actually make you more successful overall. Pick up a little trash, help the world, and help yourself!

MovieClub

Talk about a movie

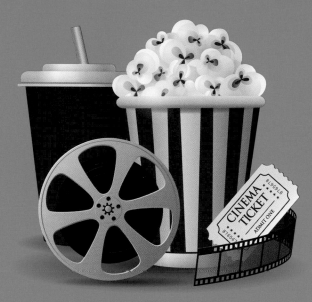

The Movie Club Challenge invites you to see a movie with friends or family members and then talk about it. Think of it like a book club, only you watch a movie instead of reading a book. Analyze the film from various perspectives—paying attention to the meaning, message, symbolism, and character development. Examine the artistic angles like cinematography, acting, music, sound, screenwriting, and story line. Most importantly, talk about how the movie made you feel and what you learned from it.

Taking time to discuss a movie with others can turn simple entertainment into a bonding, educational experience. Others will notice details and messages that you may have missed, or have insights different from your own. Even if the film doesn't meet your expectations, your group will still have a fun time, laugh together, and hopefully gain something from the discussion afterward. Turn every movie (good or bad) into a positive experience. Start planning your first movie night now!

New**Acquaintance**

Meet 4 new people

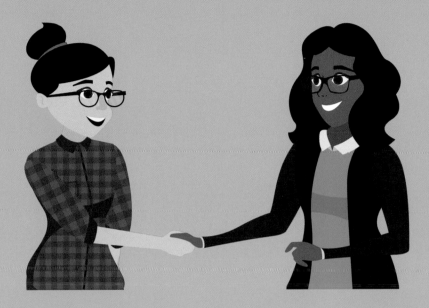

The New Acquaintance Challenge invites you to meet four new people during the next 30 days. This will be easy for some and a true challenge for others, but everyone will benefit, including the people you meet. This doesn't include meeting someone online or long distance—it needs to be in person, face to face. It sounds crazy that such a detail needs to be stipulated, but that's exactly why making a new acquaintance is important. We communicate so much electronically that we may be losing the social skills that keep us truly connected.

It can be uncomfortable meeting a new person. You may want to meet someone but think he isn't interested in talking to you. Chances are he is feeling the same way. Break the ice, introduce yourself, and ask a few questions. Your questions will show that you're interested in getting to know them and will put them at ease. Then you can enjoy having an interesting new person in your life—in the real world!

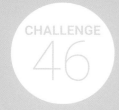

CHALLENGE
46

Old**Friend**

Reach out to an old friend

Social

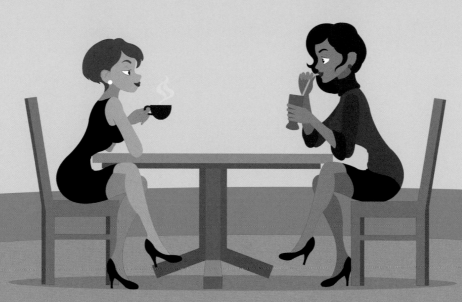

The Old Friend Challenge invites you to have a conversation with a friend whom you haven't had contact with for five years or more. Think of a friendship you cherish and take the time to rekindle that relationship. Consider someone you know who could help you in your current endeavors and use that as an excuse to reach out. It may take some work to find your friend's contact information; but with Facebook, LinkedIn, and the Internet it will probably be easier than you think.

Don't worry about what you'll talk about when you finally get together. It will be far easier than you imagine. The phrase "picking up where you last left off" is what happens with most old friends, even when they haven't talked to each other for decades. You'll have fun reliving old memories and catching up on what's happened since. You may even find ways to help each other in your current lives. Reconnecting with old friends can be nurturing, uplifting, and just plain fun!

One**World**

Learn about another culture

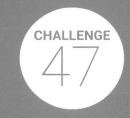

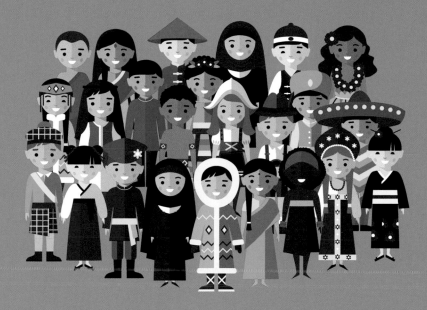

Emotional

Soc al

Occupational

The One World Challenge invites you to learn about another culture. It may be more interesting and beneficial if you choose the culture of someone you know. You can gather your research in a variety of ways: through reading, talking with someone from that culture, visiting a museum, taking a cooking class that focuses on that culture, or even watching a documentary. A combination of methods may give you the richest experience. You also get to decide when you have learned enough to call this challenge done.

Taking the time to learn about and understand others helps increase compassion and bring about acceptance. As we see life through others' eyes, we may begin to appreciate why they are the way they are and why they do the things they do. Be mindful to keep your observations at a level of compassion or admiration instead of a means to judge. Most importantly, let this newfound information propel you to look for things you have learned from the culture that you can apply to your life.

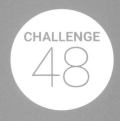

PayBack

Pay for the person behind you

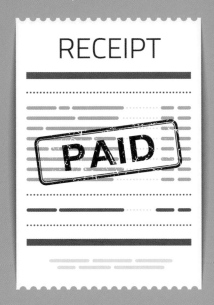

RECEIPT

PAID

The Pay Back Challenge invites you to pay for the person behind you twice in the next 30 days. You can do this when you're in line for coffee, at a drive-thru, or even at a toll booth. You could also pay for the next drink in a vending machine, or—if you're feeling generous—pay for another table at a restaurant. It doesn't have to be anonymous, but sometimes that's easier and more fun. Get creative. You only have to do it twice to complete the challenge—but hopefully you'll want to do it again and again.

Popular social theories propose that when others witness acts of generosity, like paying it back, they are more likely to do similar acts. Your single act of kindness may multiply across society like a ripple in a pond. The person you pay for may pay for the person behind them, and the cashier may even be inspired to do something similar. At a minimum, it will brighten at least one person's day. Pay it back, and make the world a better place!

PicnicBasket

Go on a picnic

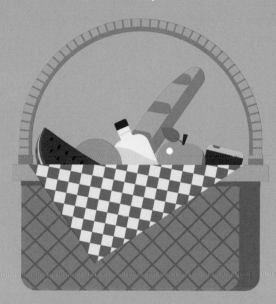

The Picnic Basket Challenge invites you to go on a picnic. Pack up some food and drinks, a blanket or tablecloth, and head for the great outdoors. Pick a place that has picnic tables like a park, lake, or campground. You could also have a picnic sitting on a blanket at the beach, on some grass, or at a scenic spot you find while hiking. You can even have a picnic in your yard! Make it a romantic date, bring your family, or invite some friends.

Picnics are like a mini vacation from regular life where you can create memories and strong bonds for everyone who gathers together. Being out in nature with others is good for your body and your soul. Fresh air is cleansing and invigorating, especially with a soothing, gentle breeze. Don't forget to bring a Frisbee or a ball. You could even try bocce, badminton, croquet, or horseshoes. Start planning your picnic: Where will you go? What will you eat? Who will you invite? It will be a fun time for everyone!

PlayNice
No teasing

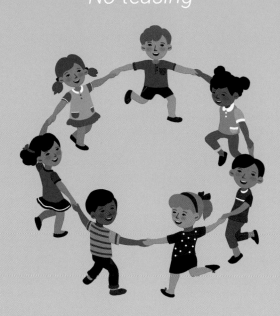

The Play Nice Challenge invites you to not tease anyone for 30 days. Remember when your parents told you that it isn't nice to tease? Well, it's still true. Many people think teasing is about having fun and trying to make people laugh. Unfortunately teasing usually points out someone else's weakness—and what's fun about that? Even if the targeted person is laughing, that doesn't mean they feel good inside. To complete this challenge, refrain from teasing for 30 days. If you slip up, apologize and call it good.

Truthfully, we tease other people to make us feel better about ourselves. Ouch! Do we really feel that badly about ourselves that we have to point out others' weaknesses to maintain our self-confidence? This may be a very hard habit to break. For some, teasing is so built into who they are, it may feel awkward to interact without teasing. Rest assured that teasing, like any other bad habit, is not part of who you are and can be changed.

SayMore

Build up another's ideas

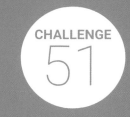

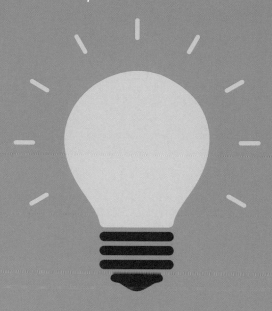

Social

The Say More Challenge invites you to help others develop their thoughts in 10 different conversations over the next 30 days. In our society, when someone makes a statement we tend to point out weaknesses of the statement instead of building on the core thought. The goal of this challenge is to encourage others to say more about their thoughts and ideas. Asking questions is a great way to encourage this. Occasionally we can also insert our own thoughts into the conversation to help build on their ideas.

You've probably heard the phrase 'no one cares how much you know until they know how much you care' (about what they know). Encouraging others to say more is a great way to show that you care enough to learn about them. In some respects, it doesn't matter what you know. You already know it. It's much more interesting to learn what others know and increase your knowledge base. Ultimately, encouraging others to say more is the first step in collaboration—combining your ideas with those of others to create new ideas.

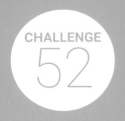
Secret007

Do 7 nice things for someone

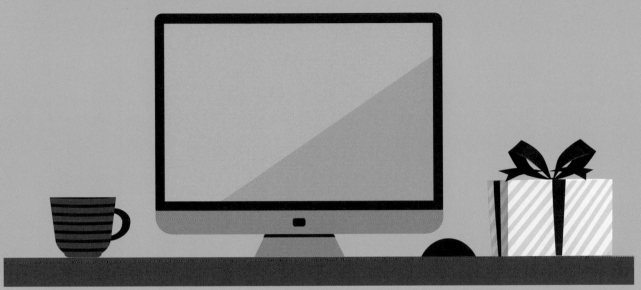

The Secret 007 Challenge invites you to do seven nice things for another person in the next 30 days without them knowing it. Big or little, noticeable or not, it will make a difference for both of you. Sneak his favorite snack onto his desk, wash her car, leave him a typed note giving him a compliment, or pull the weeds in her yard. How about putting a big bill in a tip jar, getting someone a coffee, or refraining from criticism you might normally give? Feel free to invite others to help you accomplish your kind deeds.

Focusing on other people helps you look outside of yourself, which, ironically, makes you happier. Trying to figure out what would make others happy takes it one step further. As you try to think like others do and see the world as others do, you begin to open up new horizons of understanding and it becomes easier to accept other people for who they are. (Wow! That got a little deep.) It's a lot of fun, too!

Shopping**Bag**

Use a reusable bag 6 times

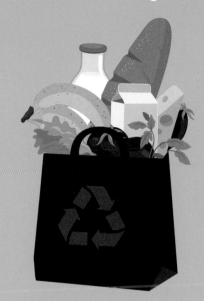

The Shopping Bag Challenge invites you to use a reusable bag at least six times over the next 30 days. If you don't already own one or more reusable bags, you can buy them for as little as a dollar each. If you don't want to purchase reusable bags, you can reuse disposable bags instead for this challenge. It's easy to remember to bring the reusable bags if you put all of them in a single bag and keep it handy in your car. When you get to the checkout line, hand your bags to the cashier. Do this for six shopping trips and you've completed the challenge.

More and more cities are charging fees for disposable shopping bags. If this trend hasn't hit your area yet, it's only a matter of time until it does. Economically and environmentally it makes a lot of sense. Why waste resources, harm wildlife, and fill landfills if you can avoid it? Also, reusable bags are generally much more sturdy and easy to handle than disposable bags. Be a team player, save some money, and help save the environment!

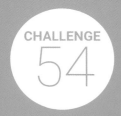
ShoutOut
30 public compliments

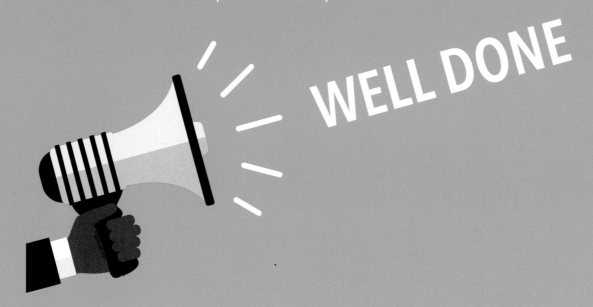

WELL DONE

The Shout Out Challenge invites you to compliment 30 people in front of others over the next 30 days. Tell the store clerk that you appreciate how friendly and fast he is. Point out something good a co-worker did during a company meeting. Praise your spouse in front of your children. Send a complimentary email to someone and copy others on the message. Aim to give at least one compliment each day during the challenge. If you forget, catch up the following day. Make sure your compliments are genuine—otherwise, it's best to say nothing.

Looking for the good in those around you will help you feel happier and more optimistic. Taking that next step to express your admiration in front of others can have a powerful positive effect for everyone who hears you. The person you compliment will be boosted by your heartfelt words. Others may chime in and confirm your compliment, giving it further strength. Giving a public compliment is like throwing a stone in a pond, creating continuous ripples of goodness that flow out into the world.

TakeIn

Bring a meal to someone

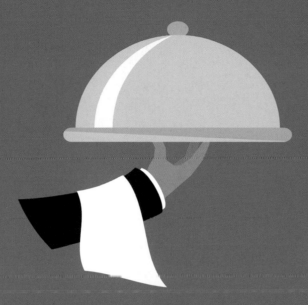

The Take In Challenge invites you to bring a meal to another person or family. Think of someone who would enjoy a home-cooked meal—someone who is sick or just had a baby, someone remodeling their kitchen, or someone who could simply use a break. Of course, take-out food is always an option, but there's nothing like a home-cooked meal. If preparing a whole meal sounds overwhelming, keep it simple. A hearty pot of soup or a pasta dish will be greatly appreciated. If the timing doesn't work for you to bring food hot, bring something they could easily warm up later.

Sometimes the challenges of life can be disheartening or exhausting. Tuning into the needs of others and offering a meal can help them nutritionally and emotionally when they see that someone else cares. Call someone today to schedule a time to take in a meal. You will fill their bellies and warm their hearts!

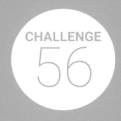

Tech Dump

Recycle electronics

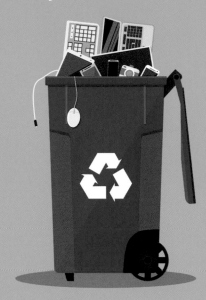

The Tech Dump Challenge invites you to recycle or donate your old, unused electronics. Check online for local options to recycle your technology waste. Some electronics stores accept e-waste at no charge and even give store credit for certain types of technology. Trash companies often accept used electronics at their waste facilities. Recycling companies also may accept used electronics. It's easy—just gather your old electronics, drop them off, and enjoy a clutter-free home!

Old electronics may contain toxic substances such as lead and mercury, which, if disposed of improperly, could be released into the environment. Also, some older electronics contain chemicals that are highly flammable and could be a fire hazard. In some areas, it's illegal to dispose of electronics with your regular trash, so resist the temptation, be a good citizen, and dispose of your electronics properly.

Un**Birthday**

Give 5 gifts

Emotional

Social

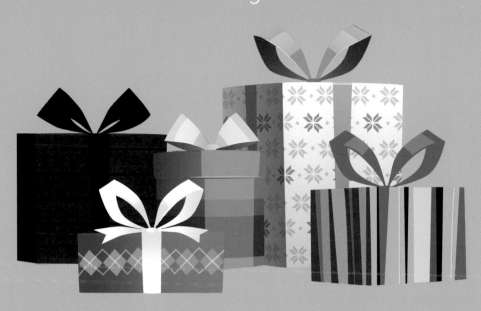

The Un Birthday Challenge invites you to give an unexpected gift to five different people over the next 30 days. Gifts for birthdays or other occasions don't count for this challenge. This way the recipient will know that the gift is from your heart, not from a sense of obligation. Try to imagine what each person would really appreciate. Spend some time with them to give you inspiration. The gift doesn't need to be expensive; it's truly the thought that counts. Bring them their favorite treat from a bakery, give them a new coffee cup, or frame a photo that they love. What matters most is that you've put some thought into it.

Gift giving is a mental exercise of looking beyond yourself to focus solely on someone else's wants, needs, and wishes, then acting upon what you discover. Giving requires your mind to shift away from your own desires to someone else's. You will develop empathy and selflessness, which will help you forget your concerns and become a happier person. It's a win–win, so get gifting!

WasteNot

Avoid disposables

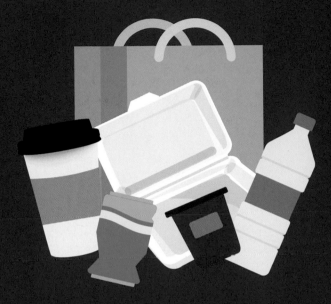

The Waste Not Challenge invites you to count how many disposable items you use in the next 30 days. Disposable products make our lives easier, but they also use up valuable resources and add to landfills. The goal of this challenge is to make you more aware of how many disposables you use each day. Hopefully, simply counting these items will encourage you to minimize their use during and after the challenge.

It's easy to reduce the number of disposable products you use. Bring your own refillable cup to the coffee shop. Carry a reusable water bottle instead of buying plastic-bottled or canned drinks. Enjoy your meals with cloth napkins. Use dish towels instead of paper towels. Store food in reusable containers instead of plastic Ziploc® bags. Choose restaurants that serve food on real plates. One of the most popular ways to meet this challenge is to bring your own reusable bags to the grocery store, or don't use any bag at all. Think of all the resources you'll save!

3Square

Eat three meals a day

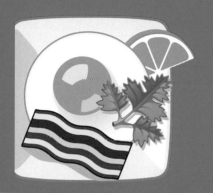 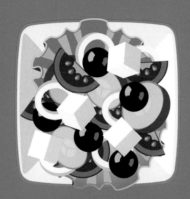 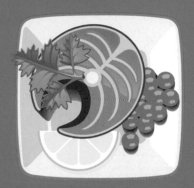

The 3 Square Challenge invites you to eat three meals a day—with no snacking in between—for 30 days. This method of eating will help you regulate how much food you eat without the complexity of counting calories. When we snack between meals or eat several small meals a day, we may never experience hunger. Hunger is actually a good thing. In fact, if you aren't hungry before your next meal, perhaps you should have eaten less at the previous meal. The opposite is also true: if you find you are hungry for hours before your next meal, you may have needed to eat more at your previous meal, including protein and good fats.

Use this as an opportunity to tune into your body. When you are hungry, embrace the sensations, knowing that you'll be completely fine until the next meal. Drink water between meals to see if you may be mistaking hunger for thirst. When you do eat, you will enjoy it even more because you will be truly hungry. Eat slowly. Savor the flavors and the experience. Sense when you've eaten just enough to fill yourself but have not overeaten to the point of feeling uncomfortable. This is a simple habit that can help you maintain your desired weight for the rest of your life!

Physical

After**Math**

Track how food makes you feel

b= brownies
c= cake
s= soda

$$3b + c + s^2 = \text{sugar crash}$$

Physical

The After Math Challenge invites you to write down what you eat and how it makes you feel each day for the next 30 days. You can eat whatever you want, as often as you want—just log it and how it makes you feel. Keep track in a journal or on your phone—something that is handy to use after you eat. If you forget to log a meal, write down what you can remember. When recording how you feel, include how full you are, your level of satisfaction, and how the food makes your body feel.

In today's busy world, we often eat on the go without giving it much thought. This simple exercise will help make you more aware of what you eat, when you eat, and how you feel afterward. Everyone's body is unique and reacts to food differently. You'll be surprised at what you learn about how different foods affect your body by simply taking a moment to notice. Hopefully this knowledge will help you to change your habits to favor foods that make you feel good—and avoid those foods that don't.

Bike100

Bike 100 miles

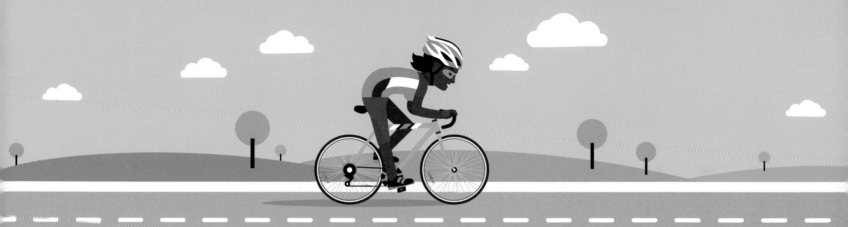

The Bike 100 Challenge invites you to ride your bicycle 100 miles over the next 30 days. This can be a really fun challenge! Ride your bike instead of taking your car. Plan rides with friends, co-workers, family, or just go solo. Choose beautiful trails or new places you'd like to see, and stop along the way to enjoy the scenery. If you don't own a bike, rent or borrow one from a friend. Always wear a helmet and bright-colored clothes for better visibility. Using a biking app can make tracking your miles easier.

Riding a bike is a healthy way to exercise, not only because of the cardio and strength benefits, but also because it puts less stress on your knees and other joints than some exercises. It also builds bone density and preserves cartilage. Cycling gives you the amazing benefit of seeing more of nature than if you were inside a car—and lets you cover more miles than if you were walking or running. Enjoy the ride!

Physical

Charge Up

Sleep without your phone

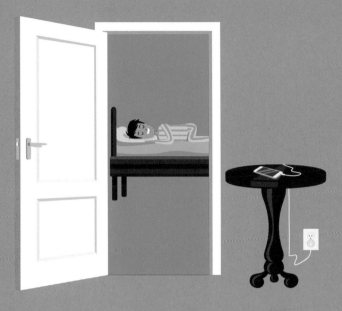

The Charge Up Challenge invites you to sleep with your cell phone in another room for 30 days. Your bedroom is an excellent place for you to recharge, but it's not the best place for charging your phone. If you use your phone as an alarm clock, find an "old school" alarm clock instead. If you're worried about missing an emergency call, leave the ringer on high so you can hear it from the other room. If you need something to do before dozing off, read a book or write in a journal—both of these evening rituals can help your mind and body relax and prepare for sleep.

Being near your cell phone at night can interfere with your ability to relax and get the rest that you need. Even if you turn off the ringer and vibration and place the phone face down to hide any light, having your phone next to your bed makes it extra tempting to check messages, browse social media, or look something up on the Internet. This can stimulate your brain when you're trying to wind down. On top of that, the light emitted from your phone mimics daylight, disrupting your body's natural sleep–wake cycles. Put your phone to rest in another room before you go to bed and get the most out of one of the great luxuries of life, sleep!

ColdShower

Take 10 cold showers

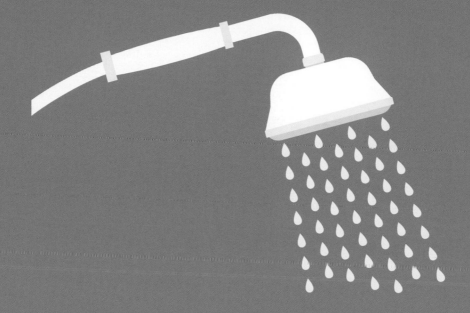

The Cold Shower Challenge invites you to brave a morning icebreaker by taking 10 cold showers in the next 30 days! This electrifying splash will invigorate you in the morning and will heighten your awareness for the rest of the day. Ease into the challenge by ending your hot shower with 15–30 seconds of cold water. Let the water spray on your feet first, then slowly move it up your body. Remain calm and breathe slowly. Your body will grow more tolerant to the cool water as the seconds pass, but if you never get past 15–30 seconds during this challenge, that's fine.

Some people feel that cold showers revive and restore our bodies. During a cold shower, you will naturally inhale more deeply and absorb more oxygen to keep you warm. Your heart rate will go up, increasing blood flow to your vital organs and creating a surge in energy. Jump into this ice water challenge—cannon ball!

FruitBasket

Keep fruit on the counter

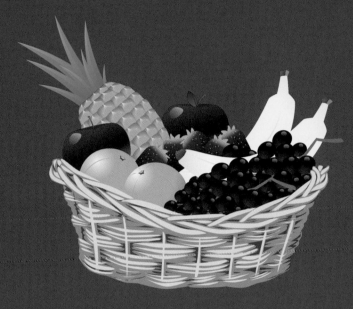

Physical

The Fruit Basket Challenge invites you to keep fruit on the counter for 30 days. Try placing it on your kitchen counter, dining table, or even somewhere in your office. Wash the fruit first—so it's ready to eat—and keep it in an attractive basket or bowl. Choose varying types of fruit, whatever is in season, since it tastes better and is usually less expensive. Before you know it, you'll be eating more fruit than ever before.

The goal of this challenge is to help you develop the habit of eating nutrient-rich fruit instead of less healthy snacks. Fruit is hydrating, packed with fiber, and contains nutrients like potassium, calcium, and antioxidants that are vital for health and healing in the body. Eating fruit can also reduce your risk of heart disease, stroke, and type-2 diabetes. It's nature's fast food!

Go**Fish**

Eat 4 servings of fish

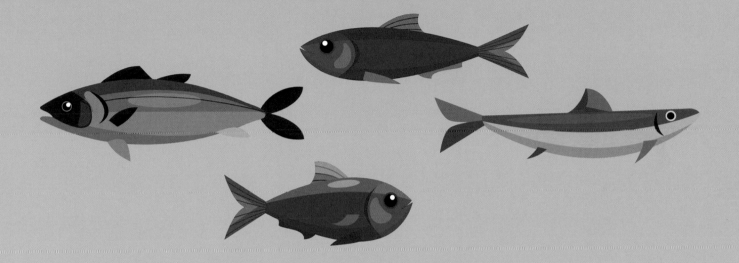

The Go Fish Challenge invites you to eat one serving (about four ounces) of fish per week for a total of four servings over the next 30 days. For this challenge it should be fish, not shellfish (lobster, crab, shrimp). If you're a vegetarian, try eating four new healthy foods that support your lifestyle. The goal of the challenge is to get you in the habit of eating fish once a week, something that most people don't do.

Fish contain many nutrients that are difficult to obtain elsewhere. They provide high-quality protein, omega-3 fatty acids, and vitamin D, most of which Americans' diets fall short. Unlike red meat, fish are low in unhealthy saturated fats. Omega-3 fatty acids are crucial for proper brain function, and they may reduce the risk of heart disease, high blood pressure, cancer, and inflammation. Tuna, mackerel, and salmon are the best fish sources of vitamin D, which most people lack during the winter months. Go fish and enhance your brainpower!

Physical

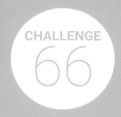

Go**Local**
Visit a farmers' market

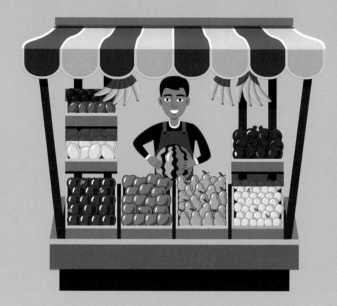

The Go Local Challenge invites you to visit a farmers' market. If you are not aware of one in your area, a quick Internet search will help. Make your trip to the farmers' market a special outing by bringing your child or a friend—or just go alone if you plan to take it slow and stay a while. The goal of the challenge is to make you aware of the fresh, nutritional, seasonal produce available at your local farmers' market in the hope that you will return.

Most of us have lost touch with how the cycles of nature relate to what we eat. We buy fruits and vegetables year-round without thinking about where they came from. At a farmers' market, you might find asparagus in the spring, sweet corn in the summer, and apples in the fall, which can help you reconnect with the earth and the seasons. Fresh-picked produce is at its peak in nutritional value and flavor. Foods you have never enjoyed before may taste new and delicious once you try them fresh from the farmers' market.

Healthy**Gut**

Try 4 probiotic foods

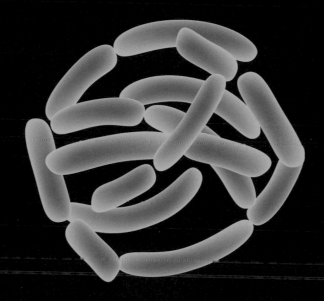

The Healthy Gut Challenge invites you to feel good from the inside out by trying four different probiotic foods during the next 30 days. While you can purchase supplements that contain probiotics, the best way to get them is from natural food sources like unsweetened yogurt, raw cheeses, pickled vegetables, sauerkraut, kimchi, kombucha, raw apple cider vinegar, brine-cured olives, kefir, and fermented soybean dishes like natto and tempeh. You can find these foods in the refrigerated section of your grocery store. Tackling this challenge can help you become more familiar with natural, probiotic-rich foods and hopefully make them a part of your regular diet.

Probiotics are active microorganisms that live in your digestive system or "gut." They are referred to as "good bacteria" because they support the immune system, reduce allergies, prevent sickness, and aid in digestion. The bacteria are naturally recurring, but today's modern diet makes it harder to keep a thriving population of good bacteria. Consciously consuming probiotic-rich foods is a good habit. It's especially important after taking antibiotics, which kill bacteria, both good and bad.

Physical

Holy**Guacamole**
Eat 10 servings of good fat

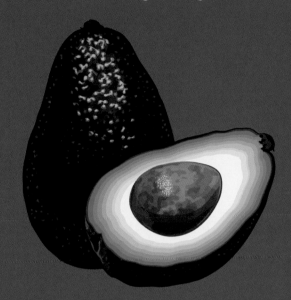

Physical

The Holy Guacamole Challenge invites you to eat 10 servings of good fat, also known as unsaturated fat during the next 30 days. You might have heard in recent studies that it's okay to eat fats again, and the goal of this challenge is to help you fit more good fats into your diet. For this challenge a good fat is defined as a whole food like avocados, olives, nuts, seeds, or fish. This does not include animal fats (except fish) or oils (even extra virgin olive oil). It's not that oils are unhealthy; they just make it easy to eat too much fat. Note your serving sizes since they're relatively small compared with other foods: 1/3 avocado, 5 olives, 24 almonds, or 4 ounces of raw fish. The goal is to encourage you to eat good foods that you might not normally eat.

It is actually healthy to eat fats because they contain essential nutrients that our body cannot produce by itself. We just need to be mindful of how much fat we eat because it has twice the calories of carbohydrates and proteins. We also need to watch out for too much animal fat and any hydrogenated fat (often found in baked goods). So enjoy some guacamole, nuts, and fish—just not too much!

Just**Dance**

Dance for 150 minutes

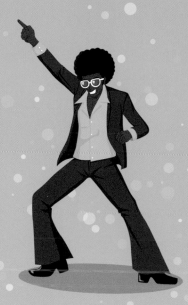

The Just Dance Challenge invites you to dance for 150 minutes during the next 30 days (an average of 5 minutes per day). Even if you're not exactly Fred Astaire, dancing can be a really fun way to exercise. You get to choose how you do the challenge. The easiest way is to turn on some music and just start dancing. Simply hearing good music will make you want to dance. Try this in the morning or when you come home from work for a quick energy boost that doesn't require workout clothes or a shower. If you like more structure, try a dance workout video, a dance app, or take a dance class. Try a night out dancing with friends for even more fun!

Dancing is a whole-body workout that's excellent for your heart, balance, and coordination. Dancing can also be a great creative outlet. You can create your own moves, choose your own music, and even dress to match the mood. Moving to the music is great for relieving stress and forgetting whatever's on your mind. Kick up your heels and just dance!

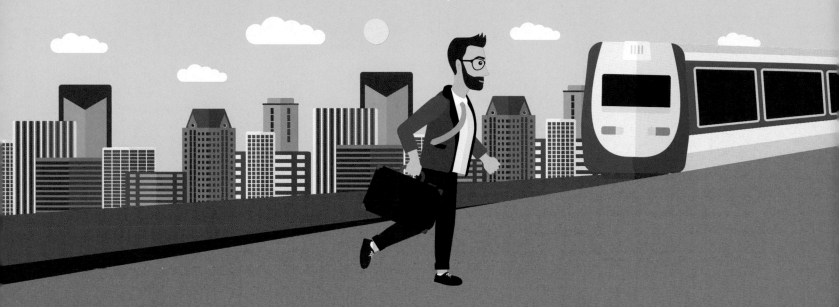

Last**Mile**

Walk part way to work

The Last Mile Challenge invites you to walk part way to work 15 out of the next 30 days. Most of us don't live within walking distance to work, but that doesn't mean that we can't walk part of the way there. If you drive to work, park a few blocks away—or at the far end of the parking lot. If you take public transportation, consider getting off at an earlier stop. Take the stairs instead of the elevator. Plan ahead so you leave home early enough to allow time for an enjoyable walk. The exact amount of walking that you add to your commute is up to you.

Walking a portion of the way to work is a simple way to add some exercise to your day—and to reap the multiple benefits it has to offer. Walking can ease joint pain, strengthen bones and muscles, boost immune function, help prevent cancer and heart disease, and keep you from gaining weight. When you walk, it gives you downtime to think and let go of stress. Walking relaxes your mind and can lighten your mood. Walking can also help you sleep better at night. Make walking part of your commute!

MeatlessMonday

No meat on Mondays

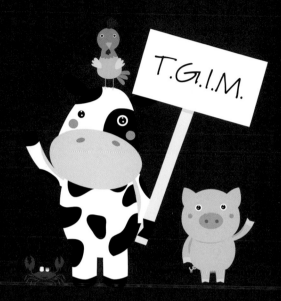

The Meatless Monday Challenge invites you to not eat any meat on Mondays for 30 days. This includes seafood, poultry, pork, and red meat. For many who feel a meal is not complete unless it includes meat, this may be quite a challenge—however, you can still have eggs and dairy. Hopefully, this challenge will get you to expand your diet and explore new, satisfying foods—even after the challenge is over. If Mondays don't work for you or if you forget one, choose whatever day of the week works best.

Meat is a great source of protein, fat, vitamins, and minerals, but too much meat can have negative effects on your health. It's also important to understand that you don't need to eat meat to live. Many cultures eat no meat at all, choosing other good sources of protein like eggs, dairy products, nuts, seeds, and legumes (beans). Another benefit of meals without meat is they tend to be less expensive and are less taxing on the environment. Take note of how your body feels after a Meatless Monday. It may be a feeling you want to have again!

Physical

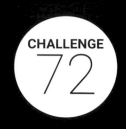

MinuteMan

Build a 72-hour kit

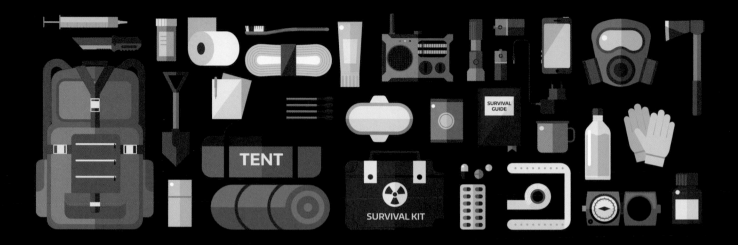

Physical

The Minute Man Challenge invites you to build a 72-hour kit. This lightweight kit contains all the food, clothing, and supplies you would need to survive for three days if you had to evacuate your home. Each person in your family should have their own kit, but for this challenge you only need to build one for yourself. If you already have one, challenge yourself to refresh your food and water supply, and confirm that your clothes still fit. You can find 72-hour kit packing lists online, but be sure to personalize it to work for your needs.

You never know when disaster might strike: hurricane, flood, or earthquake—anything that might damage your home or disrupt utilities. Having a 72-hour kit for each person in your home could be essential for you to fare well in an emergency situation. Once you have your kit assembled, store it where you can grab it quickly, if needed. It's also a good idea to inspect your kit every six months to replace food, water, or expired medications. Hopefully you'll never need your kit, but if you ever do, you'll be prepared.

Nice**Genes**

Compile a medical family tree

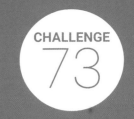

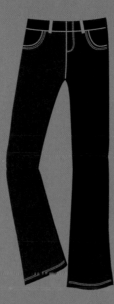

The Nice Genes Challenge invites you to compile a medical family tree. Knowing your family history can help you take the necessary precautions to prevent certain genetic conditions you may be prone to. Make a list of your grandparents, parents, uncles, aunts, siblings, children, nieces, nephews, and grandchildren. Start with those closest to you and gather the following information: gender, birthdate, ethnicity, medical conditions, mental health conditions, pregnancy complications, dates of diagnoses, alcohol and tobacco use, exercise habits, and for deceased relatives, age at death and cause of death. If that's too much for you, at least create a list of medical conditions that your parents, grandparents, and siblings have had.

Once you have your medical family tree, share it with your doctor, who can help determine preventive measures and early screenings that may apply to you. Give your medical family tree to your family, as they should also share it with their doctors. Who knows? You may save the life of a family member because you took the time to compile your family medical tree!

Physical

PearlyWhite

Use floss daily

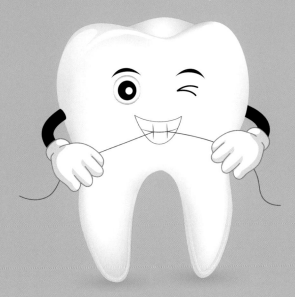

Physical

The Pearly Whites Challenge invites you to floss daily for the next 30 days. Most people brush their teeth, but many don't take the time to floss. Flossing can be awkward and unpleasant—especially if floss gets stuck between your teeth! The great thing about trying to build a habit of flossing is that brushing your teeth can be the trigger. Simply put floss next to your toothbrush as a visual reminder. After you brush in the morning or evening, floss. Over time, flossing will become as routine as brushing your teeth.

Flossing prevents plaque build-up between teeth and along the gum line, which can lead to cavities or gum disease. Simply moving the floss up in between the teeth to remove food is not enough to protect the gums. You need to also curve the floss closely around the base of each tooth and gently beneath the gum tissue. It sounds complicated, but after a few times it will be so automatic that you won't have to think about your flossing technique. Place your floss by your toothbrush and start today!

SafetyCheck

Check your smoke detector

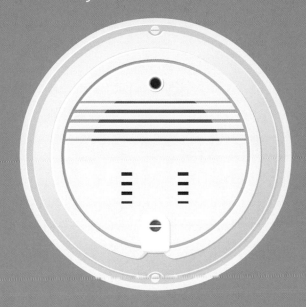

The Safety Check Challenge invites you to check the smoke detector(s) and carbon monoxide detector(s) in your home. These devices can literally save your life—unless they don't work or have a dead battery. To test most devices, press the Test button to produce a shrill sound. If there's no sound, you either need a new battery or a new device. Make sure you have both a smoke detector and a carbon monoxide detector, or a device that combines both.

For this challenge, you only need to test your safety detectors once, but it is recommended that you test them monthly. It is also recommended that you replace your batteries every six months, whether your device is battery powered or hardwired. An easy way to remember this is to do it each daylight saving time, that is, change your clocks and change your batteries. If you forget, you may hear a chirping sound or see a flashing red light on your device—this most likely means you need to replace the battery. If your devices are 10 years old or older, replace them even if they still work. Do your safety check today!

Physical

Squat 1500

50 squats a day

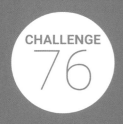
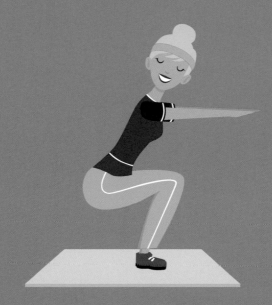

Physical

The Squat 1500 Challenge invites you to do 50 squats a day for the next 30 days. If you prefer resting your muscles for a day, do 100 squats every other day. Here are the steps to a proper squat: (1) stand with your feet spread a little wider than your hips; (2) lift your arms out straight at shoulder height; (3) start the motion by lowering your hips like you are going to sit on a chair; (4) keep shoulders back and a slight inward curve in the lower back; (5) knees should align with toes but not extend past them; (6) once you feel you are almost at chair level, squeeze the hips and return to the standing position. Check out videos online if you'd like a visual tutorial.

You may be wondering, why squats? Well, they're a great whole-body workout. When done properly, squats target several important muscle groups, including your legs and core. These are muscles you use every day for standing up, maintaining posture, and bending over. You also use these muscles when you're gardening, shoveling snow, or lifting heavy items. Keeping these muscles strong throughout your life will prevent injuries and strain. Squats also improve circulation, flexibility, and joint health. Build a daily habit of doing squats, and you'll build a healthier body for the future.

StandUp

30 standing phone calls

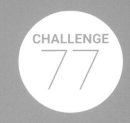

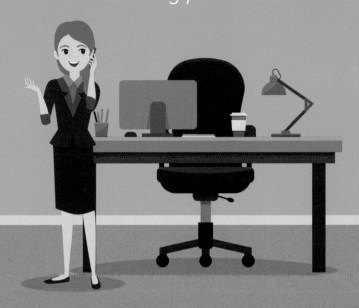

Physical

The Stand Up Challenge invites you to stand up during 30 phone calls in the next 30 days. It's that easy—just stand up when you're talking on the phone. You may want to put a note on your phone to remind you. Fortunately, most phones are cordless these days, however, if your phone is cord bound, try using speaker phone or consider getting a longer cord so you can move around more. Many office phone systems offer a mobile app so you can take office calls on your cell phone. Don't be shy. Even if you're in a room with others on a conference call, you can still stand up. They will respect you for it or maybe even join you!

Recent studies have shown that too much sitting is bad for your health, and can increase one's risk for heart disease, diabetes, stroke, and high blood pressure. It's easy to stand for a few minutes from time to time, but it may be difficult to remember to do it. This is where phone calls come in—make talking on the phone a natural trigger used to promote standing up. Once mastered, the simple habit of standing while you talk on the phone can help improve your health for the rest of your life. Next time the phone rings, stand up for your health!

TightRope

Practice balancing

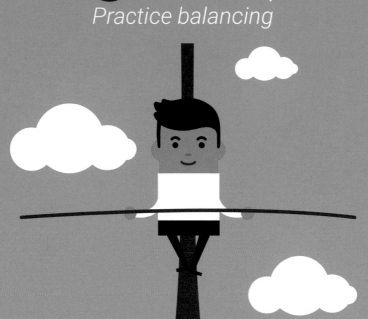

The Tight Rope Challenge invites you to spend a few minutes a day practicing your ability to balance for 20 out of the next 30 days. Pretend to walk on a tightrope by walking in a straight line, touching your heels to your toes as you walk. Feel free to guide yourself by holding a hand out along a wall or furniture while you walk. You can also practice balancing by standing on one foot at a time for a minute each. Stay by a chair or wall just in case you need some help. You may be a bit wobbly at first, but over the course of the 30 days you'll increase your stability. For a greater challenge, check out the many online resources on balance training, which offer more advanced balancing positions.

Although you probably don't associate balancing with strength training, balancing actually requires you to engage many muscle groups, particularly those in your core, legs, and back. Strengthening these muscles can help you to prevent injuries while doing daily tasks. Balancing also increases bone density and can be meditative as well—forcing you to tune in to your body. See what balancing your mind and body does for you!

Toe**Touch**

Touch your toes daily

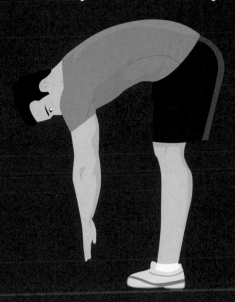

The Toe Touch Challenge invites you to spend 1–2 minutes each day trying to touch your toes for the next 30 days. Hinging at the hips, gently lean forward until you can't bend any further. Contract your abs during the motion to reduce the shear force on the lower back. Hold this position for 20–30 seconds as you feel the muscle tissue stretch. Slowly release, then repeat 3–4 times. To avoid injury, warm up your legs and lower back first by walking around briefly or even shaking out your legs a bit. If you are consistent throughout the challenge, you will see flexibility improvements.

Regular stretching can increase your range of motion and decrease your risk of injury. Stretching toward your toes lengthens your hamstrings, which can also help relieve tension in the lower back. Although touching your toes only stretches some of your muscles, it's a good start. Try incorporating additional stretches for even more benefits. Stretching can also relieve stress—breathe slowly while stretching and enjoy the release. Stay flexible by making stretching part of your daily routine!

Physical

UpBeat

500 minutes of cardio exercise

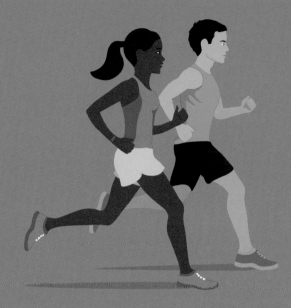

Physical

The Up Beat Challenge invites you to do 500 minutes of cardio exercise over the next 30 days—that's 125 minutes a week or 17 minutes a day. The goal of cardio exercise is to raise your heart rate for 20 minutes or more at a time. Typical cardio exercises include swimming, biking, brisk walking, running, and dancing, but you can do pretty much anything that gets your heart pumping for an extended period of time. Invite a friend to join you and make it more fun. Start with a comfortable pace and gradually increase the intensity throughout the month—if you can't talk during the exercise, are breathing too hard, or feel you're pushing too much, slow down.

Cardio exercise in the morning can be a great jumpstart to your day. Although it may sound counterintuitive, exercising actually gives you a boost of energy and releases endorphins —often called "a runner's high"—during the workout and an increase of energy throughout the day. Doing cardio doesn't just help your heart and lung health, it can also improve your mood and help you sleep better at night. Cardio exercise can even reduce your chance of getting sick. Get up and run (or bike or dance) for your life!

WaterWake-up

Drink water when you wake up

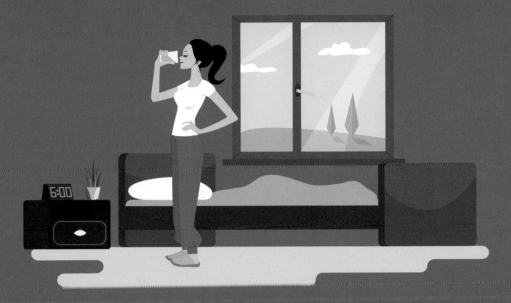

The Water Wake-up Challenge invites you to drink a glass of water when you wake up first thing in the morning for the next 30 days. If you forget, drink a glass as soon as you remember. After a long night's sleep, our bodies are typically dehydrated. A big glass of water in the morning can jumpstart your metabolism, hydrate your body, flush out toxins, and may even help you eat less. Also, you can chalk it up as your first successful accomplishment for the day!

Place a large cup of water or water bottle on your nightstand or bathroom counter each night to remind you to drink it after you wake up. Think of your body as a wilting plant that needs to be watered—rehydrating first thing in the morning will help your body perk up and perform better. Drinking 16 ounces of water is a good goal, but if that's too much for you, drink what you can. Good hydration is important for every part of your body, from your skin to your brain, so start your day right with a cup of H_2O every morning.

Physical

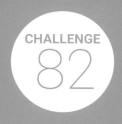

BreakTime

Take a break at work

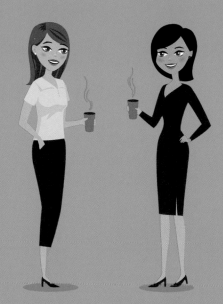

Emotional

Social

Occupational

The Break Time Challenge invites you to consciously take a break at work each day for the next 30 days. For certain jobs, breaks are mandatory and quite specifically structured, but more often than not breaks get overlooked and are considered a waste of time. In a formal setting, there's usually a 15-minute break in the morning, a 15-minute break in thc afternoon, and a 30-minute lunch break. For this challenge, you only need to take one break a day (your lunch does not count). If you miss a day, take two breaks the following day.

Breaks allow us to mentally recharge and improve our efficiency at work. The theory is that we can accomplish more in a day with breaks than in a day without breaks. If you'd like, find a break buddy and go for a walk, grab a coffee, or have a short chat. If you'd rather have time alone, read in a quiet corner or go for a walk. Another way to take a break is to switch from complex work to simple tasks like cleaning up your workspace or running an errand. Whatever style of break works for you, take one and see if you become more productive.

Certified Expert

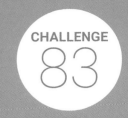

Earn a certification

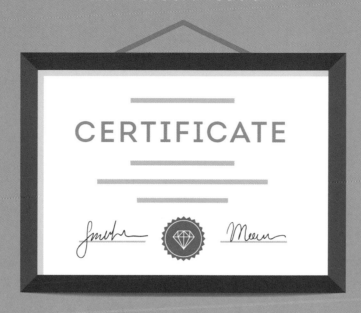

The Certified Expert Challenge invites you to earn a certification in a field related to your job or a hobby you enjoy. Some possible ideas include: education, project management, CPR, nutrition, physical fitness, software, cooking, teaching, diving, flying—the possibilities are endless. Choose something that will help you achieve your professional or personal goals. Look into your options to obtain a certification locally or online. You may even consider traveling abroad to earn your certification.

The certification process—like any type of learning—helps formalize what you know, giving you confidence to speak authoritatively on a given subject. A certification confirms that you are an expert in that field and may help you qualify for certain positions or careers. Perhaps most importantly, earning a certification gives you a sense of accomplishment and worth. What new certificate will you hang on your wall?

Occupational

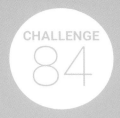
Early Bird

Arrive early

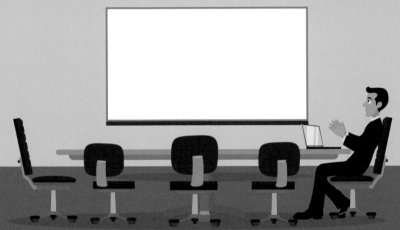

The Early Bird Challenge invites you to arrive early wherever you need to be for the next 30 days. This may sound daunting, but it's totally possible to do. If you end up arriving late or barely on time, apologize, then review what prevented you from being early and try again next time. Plan extra time just in case you run into problems with traffic or parking. When you're early, you'll probably end up waiting for other people to arrive. Take that time to prepare yourself mentally for the meeting or take a moment to clear your mind. Greet others as they arrive. Notice how you feel when the meeting begins.

Some say that being five minutes early is on time, arriving on time is late, and arriving late is unacceptable. Your punctuality sends a message to others. If you're on time, it shows that you care and respect others' time. This trust and respect flows into meetings, appointments, or social gatherings—making them much more productive and enjoyable. Strive to arrive early and see how it works for you.

Employee**Review**

Write a kind note to someone's boss

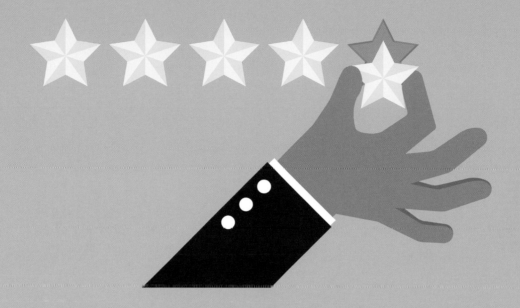

The Employee Review Challenge invites you to write a note to or speak with someone's boss about the things that person does well. It can be someone you work with or an employee at any business you frequent. It can even be a call center employee you've talked with. To complete this challenge, you only need to do this for one person. Doing this just once will make you want it to be special, not just random praise to meet a goal. Pick a person to praise who has really impressed you.

Many of us go through life noticing when people disappoint us and we feel justified in making formal complaints. Imagine what life would be like if we were to notice when people impress us and we expressed formal compliments instead. We tend to see what we aim to see. Looking for the good in others has the potential to make the world a much more enjoyable place to be. See what it does for you and the person you've praised.

Social

Occupational

FeedbackLoop

Ask 10 people for feedback

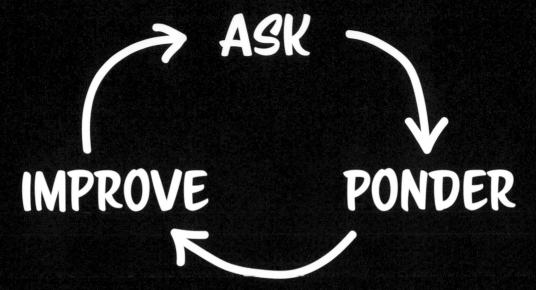

ASK

IMPROVE

PONDER

The Feedback Loop Challenge invites you to ask 10 people to tell you one thing you do well and one thing you could do better in the next 30 days. Ask people you admire, feel comfortable around, and think might have valuable insight: co-workers, friends, even family members. Be sure to listen. If you start resisting the feedback by becoming defensive or interrupting in order to explain why you do this or that, the person will likely stop providing feedback. Instead, ask questions to better understand what they are saying.

We're so close to ourselves that it's often hard to recognize our own strengths and weaknesses. Yet it is in acknowledging and understanding our strengths and weaknesses that we can grow—a desire that is an innate human attribute. Go ahead and ask for feedback. See what you learn. You can handle it. Hearing about your strengths will more than balance out your weaknesses.

Occupational

FirstPlace

Enter a contest

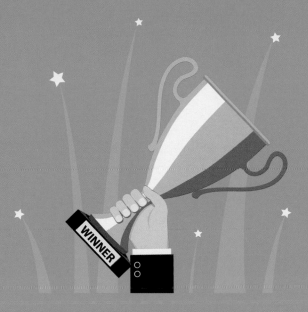

Emotional

Occupational

The First Place Challenge invites you to enter a contest. Whether or not you actually get first place isn't important—the goal of the challenge is to enter a contest, hope for the best, and enjoy the experience. Perform in a talent show or compete in a physical fitness competition. Enter a writing, photography, art, or dance contest. If you love to cook, enter a chili-feed or pie-baking contest. Check out the variety of contests offered at a county or state fair.

Participating in a contest will push you to go further, do more than you normally would, and become better at your craft. It will give you focus and drive to work on something you already enjoy. Entering a contest allows you to feel more involved. Aside from showcasing your skills at a particular craft, you might even make some new friends. Who knows, you may even win!

Job**Craft**

Redesign your job

Emotional

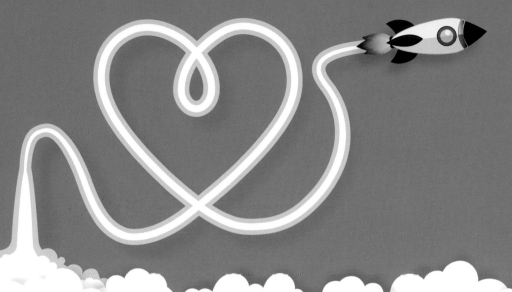

Occupational

The Job Craft Challenge invites you to change your job in a way that makes it more enjoyable for you. Of course you can't redesign your job completely, but you can make small changes to your job that can dramatically affect your job satisfaction. Work with your manager to add or remove responsibilities, change how you fulfill your responsibilities so your job incorporates one of your passions, or review how to better use your skills and abilities. Job crafting is something you can do throughout your entire career, but for this challenge you only need to craft one aspect of your job. Depending on what it is, you may or may not need to involve your manager.

Most of us spend a large portion of our lives working, so we might as well enjoy it as much as possible. Increased job satisfaction can lead to greater happiness in other areas of your life. If you're having a hard time thinking of how to change your job to make it more enjoyable, contemplate how you could do more of what you enjoy or less of what you don't enjoy. Ponder your talents and how you might use them as you work, or ask a co-worker for ideas. You won't regret it and neither will your employer!

Laser Focused

Only check email hourly

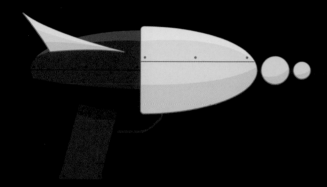

The Laser Focused Challenge invites you to resist constantly checking your email—instead, only read email once an hour for 30 days. If you'd rather make it even less frequent, like every 2 or 3 hours—it would be even better! In our age of technology and instant communication, it's easy to get into the habit of constantly responding to messages and never proactively doing anything. Step away from your email, breathe deeply, and reassure yourself that the world will not end if you don't respond to an email immediately.

We feel like we're being productive when we constantly check for messages, responding as we go, but this actually makes us less productive. Neuroscientists have found that our brains are not wired to multitask. What we really need to do is focus and concentrate on the task at hand or the people around us. Make it easier for yourself by turning off notifications on your phone and computer, then set a time to review your emails. Imagine how productive you will be with your laser focus!

Occupational

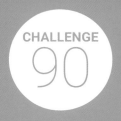

Mail**Hold**

No work emails at night

DO NOT DISTURB

The Mail Hold Challenge invites you to take a break from reading or writing work-related emails at night for 30 days. You determine if "night" means when you leave the office, after dinner, or after 8 p.m. The important thing is to set aside time at the end of the day where you can distance yourself from work. You may think continually checking in with work is a good idea, but you're actually zapping your productivity. Give yourself time away to help rejuvenate your energy and get a fresh perspective when you return to work.

Be considerate to yourself and to others. You're not the only one who needs a break in the evening. When you send an email in the evening, you may very well disrupt the recipient's evening. Sure, they could ignore your email, but it's better not to send it to them in the first place. If you think of something important that you want to act on immediately, write the email, but save it as a draft and send it the next morning. Then enjoy the rest of your evening—work free!

NetworkConnections

Meet with 5 colleagues

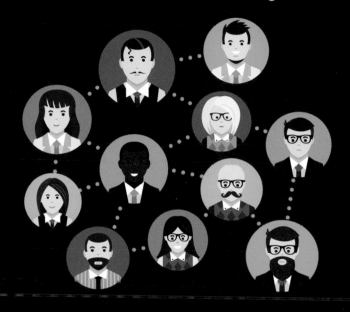

Emotional

Social

Occupational

The Network Connections Challenge invites you to meet with five colleagues (one at a time) whom you might not interact with otherwise in the next 30 days. The goal of the meeting is to better understand what they do and to get to know them better. You'll both be better for it. Your understanding of your business will grow and you will have one more resource available if you ever need help. You'll enjoy meeting with a colleague so much, it just may become a habit!

When you reach out to other people and get to know them on a personal level, magic happens. You learn things. You help each other. You introduce each other to other people. It can be a very positive experience that can help you with your job and your personal life as well. As you meet more people, your perspective will broaden and you will gain a more complete picture of your organization and the world.

Proofread|It

Check your work

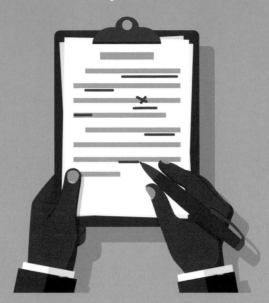

The Proofread It Challenge invites you to check over your work thoroughly before you deliver it for the next 30 days. In other words, before you send any email or share a slide deck, spreadsheet, or document, do one final review to make sure there are no mistakes. In the case of an email or any written deliverable, it's often effective to read it aloud. Try it, you'll see. Go through your work slowly as you look for errors. If you forget to do this, just remember to proofread the next one. Place a note on your desk to help you remember.

Errors can detract from your work and can even decrease the reader's confidence in you. If you don't care enough to clean up little errors, it calls into question the work itself. If you know you are weak in a particular area like spelling, grammar, or layout, have someone who is strong in that area review your work for you. This reflects well on you just as much as if you had done it yourself. Proofreading doesn't take long and it makes you look good. My editors tell me it's an easy choice to make!

¿Qué Pasa?

Learn 10 phrases in another language

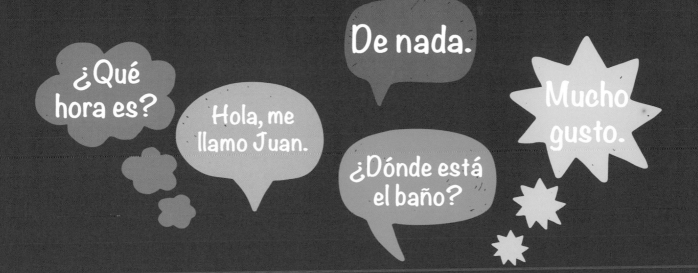

The ¿Qué Pasa? Challenge invites you to exercise your brain by learning 10 phrases in another language in the next 30 days. Choose a language that you'd like to learn—perhaps related to a place you want to visit or the language a friend speaks. Select phrases that are conversation starters, like "How are you?" and "What is your name?" or phrases that might come in handy, like "Where is the bathroom?" Good old-fashioned flash cards with the translation on the back are simple tools to help you learn. If you don't have a friend to help you with the pronunciation, listen to a recording on the Internet.

Knowing a few phrases when you travel can make a huge difference, save you time and money, and help you feel more connected to the culture. When people realize you're trying to speak their language, they are generally more accepting and willing to help you. Even if you don't plan on traveling, learning a new language will give you more efficient brain function and a better memory. Give it a try. ¡Mira qué pasa!

Occupational

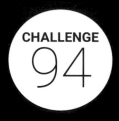

CouponClipper
Use 10 coupons

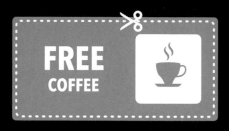

FREE
COFFEE

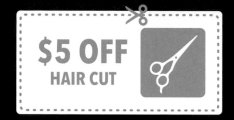

$5 OFF
HAIR CUT

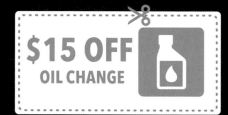

$15 OFF
OIL CHANGE

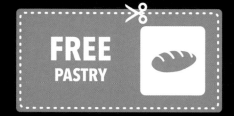

FREE
PASTRY

The Coupon Clipper Challenge invites you to use 10 coupons in the next 30 days. You can use paper coupons or digital coupons. Many grocery stores have a rewards card that gives you access to specials. Some stores have a mobile app that makes it easy to access their coupons. Don't forget to search the web for discount codes before you purchase something online. Even if you are already at the store and don't have a coupon handy, do a quick search on your cell phone for a code you can give the cashier—or ask the cashier if there are any current coupons that you can use.

More often than not, you can save some money with a coupon if you just make the effort. For many retailers, coupons are part of their business model for attracting customers. Make it part of your financial model, too! There's one caveat with coupons though: make sure you don't purchase things you don't need just because you have a coupon. Instead, stock up on items you know you'll use or only look for coupons after you've decided to buy something in particular. Get out your virtual scissors and start saving. It may take a little time, but the savings are worth it!

Financial

CreditReport

Request your free credit report

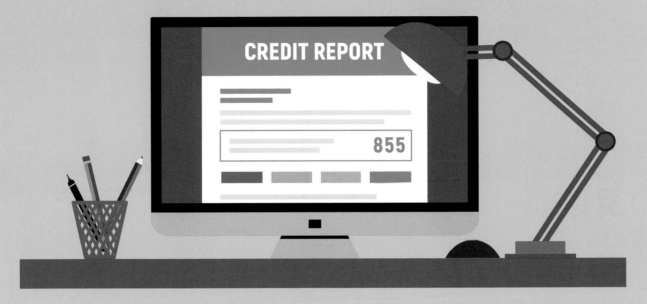

The Credit Report Challenge invites you to request a free credit report. A credit report contains the detailed information used to calculate your credit score, which is usually used to determine your eligibility for a loan or credit card or whether you qualify to rent an apartment. Many employers are now checking credit reports as part of the hiring process. Credit scores may even be used to determine your insurance premium for home and auto insurance. With so much riding on the accuracy of your credit report, it's important that the information in it is correct!

To request your free credit report, go to AnnualCreditReport.com. You will then select one of the three credit reporting agencies: Equifax, Experian, or TransUnion. You can request your report from each of the agencies once each year—you can stagger your requests and check a different one every four months. For this challenge, you only need to request one credit report. When you get it, review it carefully for inaccuracies. If you find any, the credit report will contain instructions on how to dispute errors. Take this important step to financial stability and request your free credit report today!

Financial

EmergencyFund

Create a bank account for emergencies

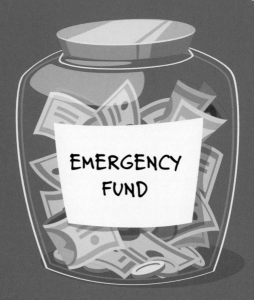

The Emergency Fund Challenge invites you to create a separate bank account for emergencies. Call your bank, ask them to set up a new savings account, move some money into it, and you're done! It's that easy. The amount you put into the account is up to you. (But watch out for minimum balance requirements to avoid fees!) Start with enough funds to cover a surprise auto repair or similar spending emergency. If that's more than you have, start with any amount and set up regular deposits. Financial experts recommend that an emergency fund contain enough to live on for three to six months, but this challenge only asks that you open a separate account and deposit any amount to get started.

An emergency fund can help you avoid going into debt when a financial surprise occurs in your life. Typically, sudden unexpected purchases lead to credit card debt or payment plans, which end up costing you more money because of the high interest rates. Having an emergency fund in a separate account ensures that the money is readily available and not needed for monthly bills. Once your emergency fund is set up, make sure to resist the temptation to use it to purchase something that's not an emergency!

Estate**Planning**

Create a will

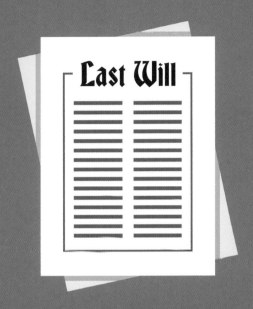

The Estate Planning Challenge invites you to create a will. If you already have a will, review it and see if you'd like to make any changes. If you don't have a will, now is a great time to make one! You can create your will under the guidance of an estate attorney or through a legal online website. There are several important decisions to make as you write your will. You'll need to select your beneficiaries and the executor of your will. If you have children who are minors or dependents, you must choose a guardian for them (and ask the friend or family member if they will accept that responsibility).

Next, assess your property and decide who gets what. You can list what percentage of your total assets goes to each beneficiary or you can specify exactly what each person will inherit. Your attorney or legal website can guide you through the technicalities. Once you've completed your will, store it somewhere safe and let your executor know where to find it. It may not be something you want to face, but if you don't have a will when you die, a court will make the decisions for you—most likely not in the way you would have chosen.

Financial

98

Fine-Tooth**Comb**
Review your bills

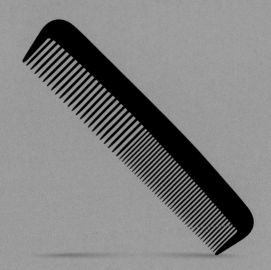

The Fine-Tooth Comb Challenge invites you to review all your bills for one month. Go through each bill slowly to make sure you understand every charge and that you are still using the specific service for which you are paying. If a charge doesn't make sense, call and ask for an explanation. Don't forget to review the charges on your credit card bills to confirm each charge is valid. You can also check to see if returns are properly credited on your account. If you use autopay, log in to the biller's website and review the bill online.

Going paperless is a great idea, but can often cause us to overlook specifics on bills. You may be surprised at how many charges are actually there. You may discover that you forgot to cancel a free trial or there may have been a price hike for a monthly service. You can also identify ways to cut back on services, utilities, or purchases. Reviewing your bills doesn't take much effort, but can have great returns!

Financial

MoneyBuddy

Check-in for purchases over $50

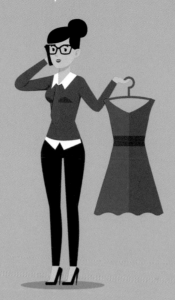

The Money Buddy Challenge invites you to check in with your spouse, trusted friend, or significant other before making any purchases over $50 for the next 30 days. Being accountable to someone for any expenditures over $50 will help you think twice before spending—a good habit to have. It's easy. Select a money buddy and explain the challenge to them. Then, before you make a purchase over $50, call or text your buddy. Once they've confirmed it is not a hastily made or imprudent decision, go ahead with the purchase.

This system may delay the process of making purchases, but that's a good thing when it comes to finances. Marketers do all they can to promote impulse purchases, and even though some impulse purchases do end up being sound, many aren't things we actually need. Having a money buddy to authorize your purchases can be a very effective way to limit poor purchases—keeping more money in your wallet. It may be a bit awkward initially, but it works and can be a lot of fun! Give it a try.

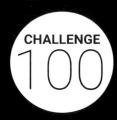

Money**Fast**

No spending money for 4 days

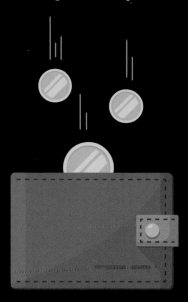

The Money Fast Challenge invites you to not spend any money during four out of the next 30 days. You pick the days and they don't need to be consecutive, unless you want a real challenge! Perhaps you can pick the same day each week. Your spending freeze includes online purchases, eating out, gas, groceries, etc. If you have to pay a toll or buy a bus pass that you can't pay for in advance, that's fine. Otherwise, make a point to plan ahead or go without.

You may be wondering what difference it makes to purchase things a day earlier or a day later. The goal of this challenge is to increase spending awareness. On the day you are not spending any money, you will become very aware of what you normally spend it on. This awareness can help you better prioritize wants and needs. When you plan ahead you will likely spend more efficiently, that is, when you wait to spend money you will tend to spend less. Give it a try—it's only four days. See what a money fast can do for your spending habits!

Financial

Piggy**Bank**
Visit with a financial advisor

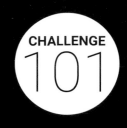

CHALLENGE
101

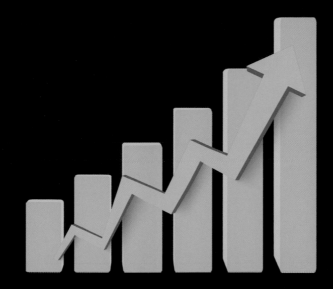

The Piggy Bank Challenge invites you to meet with a financial advisor or, if you already have one, to set up a meeting with your advisor to see if any adjustments should be made to your investment strategy—something you should do at least annually. If you don't have a financial advisor, ask your friends or colleagues for recommendations. If you already have money invested through work or otherwise, contact the brokerage and ask to speak with an advisor. If you don't have a brokerage, most brokerages are happy to connect you with an advisor.

A financial advisor is someone who can help you plan for your future financial needs—like your children's college expenses and your retirement. They have tools to help you calculate how much money you should be saving to meet your goals. They can help guide you as to which investment tools could best maximize your tax advantages and which types of investments best match your risk tolerance. They are experts in a field that you may not understand as well. Reach out to a financial advisor today and be ready for tomorrow!

Financial

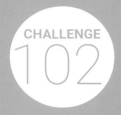

Social **Security**

Create a Social Security account

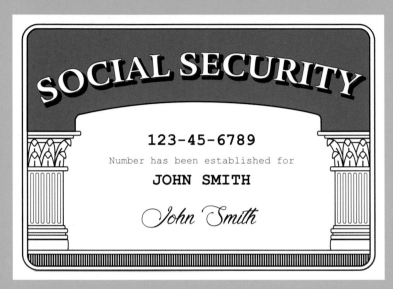

The Social Security Challenge invites you to create an account with the Social Security Administration. Go to ssa.gov to create your online account. You need to be at least 18 years old and have your social security number, an email address, and a physical mailing address. It's that easy to complete this challenge. You'll be done in minutes.

With your Social Security online account, you'll be able to see your estimated benefits at retirement, disability benefits, and dependent benefits upon your death. You will also be able to review your lifetime earnings history and get information about Medicare eligibility and benefits. All this information will be useful as you plan for your retirement—and it's fun to read since it's all about the money that will be paid to you!

Financial